NO GALLBLADDER DIET COOKBOOK

100+ Delicious Recipes to Help You Stay Healthy and Satisfied After Gallbladder Surgery

LOIS R. WALKER

CONTENTS

INTRODUCTION 5

UNDERSTANDING THE NO GALLBLADDER DIET 6

Essential Tips for Cooking and Eating 7

Food to Avoid and to Include 9

Breakfast Recipes...11

Oatmeal with Berries and Almonds...............11

Greek Yogurt Parfait 12

Smoothie Bowl..13

Scrambled Eggs with Spinach and Tomatoes 14

Whole Wheat Toast with Avocado and Poached Egg 15

Quinoa Breakfast Bowl 16

Cottage Cheese Pancakes 17

Vegetable Frittata 18

Chia Seed Pudding.......................................19

Banana Almond Butter Toast.......................20

Egg Muffins...21

Yogurt and Fruit Smoothie 22

Vegetable Omelette 23

Buckwheat Pancakes....................................24

Salmon and Avocado Toast..........................25

Fruit and Nut Breakfast Bowl 26

Vegetable Breakfast Burrito 27

Peanut Butter Banana Smoothie...................28

Egg and Veggie Breakfast Casserole 29

Lunch Recipes...30

Grilled Lemon Herb Chicken Salad 30

Quinoa and Vegetable Stir-Fry......................31

Salmon and Avocado Wrap 32

Turkey and Hummus Veggie Wrap................33

Mediterranean Chickpea Salad 34

Vegetable and Lentil Soup 36

Tuna and White Bean Salad..........................37

Grilled Veggie and Chicken Kabobs 38

Shrimp and Avocado Salad 39

Vegetable and Turkey Sauté 40

Dinner Recipes...41

Grilled Lemon Herb Chicken with Steamed Vegetables 41

Turkey and Vegetable Stir-Fry.......................42

Baked Cod with Lemon Garlic Butter Sauce and Steamed Green Beans...............................43

Shrimp and Veggie Skewers with Brown Rice 44

Baked Salmon with Quinoa and Roasted Asparagus..45

Vegetarian Chili with Whole Grain Bread.......46

Tofu Stir-Fry with Brown Rice.......................47

Grilled Chicken Caesar Salad 48

Quinoa Stuffed Bell Peppers 49

Vegetable and Chickpea Curry with Cauliflower Rice..50

Snacks 51

Greek yogurt with berries 51

Hummus with sliced vegetables 52

Apple slices with almond butter 53

Cottage cheese with pineapple 54

Edamame...55

Trail mix 56

Appetizers 57

Grilled Vegetable Skewers 57

Hummus with Veggie Sticks 58

Caprese Salad Skewers 59

Cucumber Roll-Ups 60

Stuffed Mushrooms............................. 61

Shrimp Cocktail................................... 62

Guacamole with Baked Tortilla Chips 63

Quinoa Stuffed Peppers..................... 64

Cucumber Tomato Salad Cups.................... 65

Soup & Stew.. 66

Chicken and Vegetable Soup..................... 66

Butternut Squash Soup........................ 67

Turkey Chili....................................... 68

Vegetable Lentil Soup......................... 69

Tomato Basil Soup 70

Potato Leek Soup 71

Minestrone Soup................................. 72

Vegetable Quinoa Soup....................... 73

Mushroom Barley Soup 74

Poultry 75

Grilled Lemon Herb Chicken Breast.............. 75

Baked Pesto Chicken Thighs 76

Slow Cooker Chicken and Vegetable Stew 77

Chicken and Vegetable Stir-Fry 78

Grilled Honey Mustard Chicken Skewers 79

Baked Chicken Parmesan 80

Lemon Garlic Chicken Pasta................. 81

Chicken and Vegetable Curry 82

Chicken Caesar Salad Wraps 83

Fish & Seafood.................................... 84

Poached Salmon with Lemon Dill Sauce 84

Tilapia 85

Poached Cod with Tomato and Basil:........... 86

Baked Trout with Lemon and Herbs 87

Poached Trout with Lemon and Dill.............. 88

Sardines... 89

Poached Mackerel with Vegetables.............. 90

Shrimp Base 91

Baked Scallops with Garlic and Parmesan 92

Flounder... 93

Haddock Poached in Tomato Broth.............. 94

Desserts... 95

Fruit Salad.. 95

Baked Apples 96

Greek Yogurt Parfait............................ 97

Chia Seed Pudding 98

Banana Nice Cream 99

Rice Pudding...................................... 100

Coconut Macaroons 101

Pumpkin Pie Smoothie 102

Oatmeal Cookies................................ 103

Angel Food Cake with Berries 104

MEAL PLANNING 105

Frequently Asked Questions (FAQs)........... 107

GLOSSARY 108

INTRODUCTION

The "No Gallbladder Diet Cookbook" is a comprehensive guide to nourishing meals for optimal digestive health, and it is our pleasure to introduce it to you.

Even though living without a gallbladder might provide its own set of obstacles, it is possible to continue to enjoy tasty and gratifying meals while also supporting good digestive health if you make the appropriate dietary choices. When it comes to assisting persons who have had gallbladder removal surgery, the "No Gallbladder Diet Cookbook" serves as your go-to resource, giving a broad assortment of dishes that are specifically designed to benefit those folks.

To educate you with information about the function of the gallbladder in digestion, the adaptations your body takes following its removal, and the dietary practices that might promote your well-being, this cookbook goes beyond just giving recipes. Its goal is to empower you with knowledge. Whether you are a patient who has just had surgery or have been living without a gallbladder for a considerable amount of time, this cookbook will meet your nutritional requirements by providing you with a wide range of alternatives that are both savory and healthy.

The contents of this book include a plethora of recipes that have been developed to be kind to your digestive system, hence reducing the possibility that you may experience pain or digestive distress. Every single food has been carefully crafted to cater to the requirements of those who are adjusting to a life without a gallbladder. This includes soups that are light and easy to digest, salads that are filled with nutrients, robust main courses, and desserts that are very delicious.

In addition, the cookbook provides useful advice on how to substitute ingredients, reduce portion sizes, and engage in mindful eating activities to further improve your digestive experience. On your road toward a diet that does not need a gallbladder, this cookbook is an invaluable companion. Whether you are looking to control your weight, improve your general health, or just find inspiration for preparing delicious meals without sacrificing the comfort of your digestive system, this cookbook comes highly recommended.

You may give yourself more power by using the information and culinary creativity that can be found in the "No Gallbladder Diet Cookbook." Say goodbye to dull and limiting meals, and embrace a broad assortment of foods that not only help your digestive system but also provide delight to your eating experience. Let this cookbook be your guide to enjoying a vivid and rewarding culinary journey suited to your nutritional requirements.

UNDERSTANDING THE NO GALLBLADDER DIET

The no gallbladder diet, also known as the post-cholecystectomy diet, is a food plan meant to assist persons who have had their gallbladder removed to control their digestion and reduce pain. The gallbladder is an organ that stores bile generated by the liver and releases it to help in the digestion of lipids. When the gallbladder is removed, bile is continually discharged into the digestive system, which may occasionally lead to digestive difficulties, particularly with fatty meals.

Here are some major components of the no-gallbladder diet:

1. Low-fat meals: Since the gallbladder aids in digesting fats, persons lacking a gallbladder may have difficulties digesting high-fat foods. Therefore, it's advisable to take low-fat or lean choices. This includes items like lean meats, chicken without skin, fish, low-fat dairy products, and plant-based sources of protein.

2. Moderate consumption of good fats: While high-fat meals should be avoided, it's still vital to have healthy fats in the diet for general health. Healthy fats may be found in foods like avocados, almonds, seeds, and olive oil. However, it's vital to take them in moderation to prevent overloading the digestive system.

3. Fiber-rich foods: Fiber may help regulate digestion and reduce constipation, which can be a frequent concern following gallbladder surgery. Incorporate lots of fruits, vegetables, whole grains, and legumes into your diet to guarantee a sufficient intake of fiber.

4. Small, frequent meals: Instead of huge meals, opt for smaller, more frequent meals throughout the day. This may assist smooth the digestion process and avoid overloading the system with a huge quantity of food at once.

5. Avoid trigger foods: Certain foods may increase digestive issues in those without a gallbladder. These may include fatty or fried meals, spicy foods, caffeine, carbonated drinks, and alcohol. It's vital to pay attention to how your body responds to various meals and avoid those that cause pain.

6. Stay hydrated: Drinking enough water is vital for general digestion and may help avoid constipation, which is common after gallbladder surgery. Aim to drink at least 8 glasses of water every day, and more if you're physically active or live in a hot region.

7. Gradually reintroduce foods: After surgery, it may take some time for your digestive system to adapt. Start with bland, easily digested meals and gradually reintroduce more foods into your diet while paying attention to how your body reacts.

ESSENTIAL TIPS FOR COOKING AND EATING

Cooking and eating on a no-gallbladder diet might be feasible with some tweaks to your culinary practices. Here are crucial guidelines to assist you manage cooking and eating after gallbladder removal:

1. Choose lean proteins: Opt for lean protein sources such as skinless chicken, fish, and lean cuts of meat, tofu, and lentils. Avoid frying and pick healthy cooking techniques like baking, grilling, steaming, or sautéing with less oil.

2. Limit saturated and trans fats: Reduce your consumption of saturated and trans fats, which might be tougher to digest. This includes avoiding deep-fried meals, processed snacks, and fatty types of meat. Instead, concentrate on adding healthy fats like olive oil, avocados, and almonds in moderation.

3. Monitor portion sizes Instead of eating huge meals, split your daily food consumption into smaller, more regular meals. This helps avoid overloading your digestive system and encourages healthier digestion.

4. Include soluble fiber: Soluble fiber may aid with digestion and control bowel motions. Include foods high in soluble fiber, such as oats, barley, fruits, vegetables, and legumes. However, increase fiber gradually to enable your digestive system to acclimate.

5. Stay hydrated: Drinking adequate water is vital for digestion and general health. Aim to eat lots of water throughout the day, and consider sipping fluids between meals to prevent overloading your digestive system during meals.

6. Moderate usage of spices: While spicy meals may be accepted by some, others may find them annoying. Experiment with light spices and herbs to improve taste without creating pain. Pay attention to your body's responses and adjust your spice levels appropriately.

7. Experiment with low-fat cooking techniques: Explore cooking techniques that utilize less fat, such as baking, grilling, broiling, steaming, and poaching. These approaches may help you enjoy tasty dishes without sacrificing taste.

8. Choose readily digested foods: Initially, concentrate on readily digested meals such as cooked vegetables, well-cooked grains, and easily digestible meats. As your body adapts, you may gradually reintroduce a range of foods.

9. Limit processed and high-sugar foods: Processed and high-sugar meals may induce stomach pain. Focus on complete, nutrient-dense meals and restrict your consumption of processed snacks, sweets, and sugary drinks.

10. Keep a food diary: Track what you consume and write any symptoms or discomfort. This may help you discover trigger foods and adapt your diet appropriately. Share this information with your healthcare physician or dietician for specific recommendations.

11. Consider digestive enzymes: Some persons find comfort in taking digestive enzyme supplements with meals to help in the breakdown of lipids. Consult with your healthcare practitioner before adding supplements to your routine.

Remember that everyone's tolerance to certain meals differs, so it's crucial to listen to your body and make modifications depending on your specific requirements. If you have particular concerns or questions regarding your diet after gallbladder ectomy, talk with a healthcare provider or a certified dietitian for individualized counsel.

FOOD TO AVOID AND TO INCLUDE

After gallbladder removal, it's vital to make dietary modifications to decrease digestive pain and maintain general health. Here are things to avoid and incorporate into a no gallbladder diet:

Foods to Avoid

1. High-fat foods: These might be difficult to digest without the gallbladder. Avoid things like fried dishes, fatty cuts of meat, high-fat dairy items, and creamy sauces.

2. Spicy foods: Spicy meals may irritate the digestive system and create pain. Limit or avoid meals seasoned with hot peppers, chili powder, or other spicy substances.

3. Highly processed foods: Processed meals, particularly those heavy in harmful fats and chemicals, may be taxing on the digestive system. Avoid goods like fast meals, packaged snacks, and processed meats.

4. Carbonated beverages: Carbonated drinks may produce bloating and gas, which may be painful for some persons following gallbladder removal.

5. Caffeinated beverages: Caffeine may irritate the digestive system and produce discomfort. Limit or avoid caffeinated liquids like coffee, tea, and soda.

6. Alcohol: Alcohol may be demanding on the liver and may worsen digestive difficulties. Limit or avoid alcoholic drinks, particularly if they cause pain.

7. Certain raw vegetables: Some raw vegetables, such as cabbage, broccoli, cauliflower, and onions, might be difficult to stomach for some individuals. Cook these veggies thoroughly to make them simpler to digest.

8. High-sugar foods: Sugary meals and drinks may interrupt digestion and may lead to digestive pain. Limit your consumption of sweets, sugary snacks, and sugary beverages.

Foods to Include

1. Lean proteins: Choose lean protein sources such as skinless chicken, fish, tofu, lentils, and lean cuts of meat like pork loin or beef sirloin.

2. Low-fat dairy: Opt for low-fat or fat-free dairy products such as skim milk, yogurt, and cheese to limit fat consumption.

3. Healthy fats: Include sources of healthy fats such as avocados, nuts, seeds, and olive oil in moderation.

4. Whole grains: Choose whole grains like brown rice, quinoa, oats, and whole wheat bread to enhance fiber intake and support good digestion.

5. Fruits and vegetables: Incorporate a variety of fruits and vegetables into your diet, concentrating on those that are readily digested. Cooked or steamed veggies may be friendlier on the digestive tract than raw ones.

6. Fiber-rich foods: Include fiber-rich meals like beans, lentils, chickpeas, fruits, and vegetables to promote digestive health and avoid constipation.

7. Hydration: Drink lots of water throughout the day to keep hydrated and help digestion. Aim for at least eight glasses of water daily, and more if you're physically active or live in a hot region.

8. Digestive aids: Consider introducing digestive aids such as probiotics or digestive enzyme supplements to improve digestion, but speak with a healthcare practitioner before doing so.

Remember that individual tolerance to different meals may vary, so it's crucial to pay attention to how your body responds to certain foods and alter your diet appropriately. If you're unclear about what foods to include or avoid, consider talking with a qualified dietitian for tailored assistance.

BREAKFAST RECIPES

Oatmeal with Berries and Almonds

Cooking Time: 5 minutes | **Prep Time**: 5 minutes | **Total Time**: 10 minutes | **Servings**: 1

Ingredients:

- 1/2 cup rolled oats
- 1 cup water or unsweetened plant-based milk (almond, oat, etc.)
- 1/4 cup fresh or frozen berries (blueberries, raspberries, strawberries, etc.)
- 1/4 cup sliced almonds
- 1/2 teaspoon ground cinnamon (optional)
- 1/4 teaspoon ground ginger (optional)
- Honey or maple syrup to taste (optional)

Directions:

1. In a saucepan, combine oats and water or plant-based milk. Bring to a boil over medium heat, then reduce heat and simmer for 5 minutes, or until oats are cooked through and creamy.
2. Remove from heat and stir in berries, almonds, cinnamon, and ginger (if using).
3. Let cool slightly before serving.
4. Drizzle with honey or maple syrup to taste (optional).

Nutrition Information: Calories: 350, Fat: 8g, Cholesterol: 0mg, Sodium: 130mg, Carbohydrates: 50g, Fiber: 8g, Protein: 6g

Tips:

- For a thicker oatmeal, use less water or milk.
- You can substitute other nuts or seeds for the almonds, such as walnuts, pecans, or chia seeds.
- Add a scoop of protein powder for an extra boost of protein.
- Get creative with the toppings! Other options include chopped fruit, shredded coconut, or a drizzle of nut butter.

Greek Yogurt Parfait

Cooking time: 5 minutes | **Prep time**: 5 minutes | **Total time**: 10 minutes | **Serving** size: 1

Ingredients:

- 1/2 cup plain Greek yogurt
- 1/4 cup sliced strawberries
- 1/4 cup blueberries
- 1/4 cup chopped banana
- 1/4 cup granola (choose a low-fat, low-sugar variety)
- 1 tablespoon chopped nuts (optional)
- 1/4 cup poached pear, sliced (optional)
- 1 tablespoon honey or maple syrup (optional)

Directions:

1. If using, poach the pear: Bring a small pot of water to a simmer. Add the pear and simmer for 5-10 minutes, or until tender. Drain and cool.
2. In a serving glass, layer the yogurt, strawberries, blueberries, banana, granola, nuts (if using), and poached pear (if using).
3. Drizzle with honey or maple syrup (if using).
4. Serve immediately.

Nutrition information: Calories: 250, Fat: 5g, Saturated fat: 2g, Cholesterol: 5mg, Sodium: 80mg, Carbohydrates: 30g, Fiber: 5g, Sugar: 15g, Protein: 20g

Tips:

- You can use any type of fruit that you like in this parfait.
- If you are looking for a more filling parfait, you can add a scoop of protein powder to the yogurt.
- Make sure to choose a low-fat, low-sugar granola to keep this parfait healthy.
- If you don't have time to poach a pear, you can use canned pears that have been drained and rinsed.
- You can also add a sprinkle of cinnamon or nutmeg to the parfait for extra flavor.

Smoothie Bowl

Prep Time: 5 minutes | **Cooking Time:** 0 minutes | **Total Time:** 5 minutes | **Serving Size:** 1

Ingredients:

- 1 cup unsweetened plant-based milk (almond, soy, oat, etc.)
- 1/2 frozen banana
- 1/4 cup frozen berries (mixed, blueberries, raspberries, etc.)
- 1 scoop plant-based protein powder (optional)
- 1/2 tablespoon ground flaxseed or chia seeds
- 1/4 teaspoon cinnamon
- Pinch of nutmeg

Optional Toppings:

- Fresh berries
- Sliced banana
- Chopped nuts or seeds
- Granola (choose low-fat, low-sugar options)
- Unsweetened shredded coconut

Directions:

1. Blend all ingredients together in a blender until smooth and creamy. Adjust the consistency by adding more or less milk.
2. Pour the smoothie into a bowl.
3. Top with your desired toppings.

Nutrition Information: Calories: 250-350, Fat: 5-10g, Carbs: 30-40g, Fiber: 5-10g, Protein: 10-20g

Tips:

- Choose low-fat ingredients, such as unsweetened plant-based milk and protein powder.
- Avoid fatty fruits, such as avocados and mangoes.
- Limit added sugars and artificial sweeteners.
- Use ground flaxseed or chia seeds for added fiber and healthy fats.
- Listen to your body and adjust the recipe as needed based on your individual tolerance.

Scrambled Eggs with Spinach and Tomatoes

Cooking Time: 10 minutes | **Prep Time**: 5 minutes | **Total Time**: 15 minutes | **Serving Size**: 1

Ingredients:

- 2 eggs
- 1 tablespoon unsweetened almond milk or low-fat milk
- 1/4 teaspoon olive oil
- 1/2 cup chopped spinach
- 1/4 cup chopped cherry tomatoes
- Salt and pepper to taste
- Optional: Chopped fresh herbs like parsley or chives

Directions:

1. Whisk together the eggs and milk in a bowl. Season with a pinch of salt and pepper.
2. Heat the olive oil in a non-stick pan over medium heat.
3. Add the spinach and cook until wilted, about 1 minute.
4. Pour in the egg mixture and scramble until just set, about 2-3 minutes.
5. Stir in the tomatoes and cook for another minute, or until heated through.
6. Remove from heat and season with additional salt and pepper, to taste.
7. Serve immediately, garnished with fresh herbs if desired.

Nutrition Information: Calories: 220, Protein: 18g, Fat: 10g, Carbohydrates: 5g, Fiber: 1g, Cholesterol: 210mg, Sodium: 180mg

Tips:

- Use low-fat or fat-free milk instead of almond milk if preferred.
- Add other vegetables like chopped bell peppers or mushrooms.
- Serve on whole-wheat toast or with a side of fruit.
- For a richer flavor, use a small amount of grated Parmesan cheese.
- Make sure to not overcook the eggs, as they can become tough and rubbery.
- If you have any concerns about following a no gallbladder diet, it's important to consult with a registered dietitian or other healthcare professional.

Whole Wheat Toast with Avocado and Poached Egg

Cooking Time: 10 minutes | **Prep Time**: 5 minutes | **Total Time**: 15 minutes | **Serving Size**: 1

Ingredients:

- 2 slices whole wheat bread
- 1/2 ripe avocado, mashed
- 1 egg
- 1 tablespoon apple cider vinegar or white vinegar
- Salt and pepper to taste
- Optional toppings: sliced cherry tomatoes, fresh herbs (like cilantro or chives), hot sauce

Directions:

1. Toast the bread: Toast the bread in a toaster to your desired level of crispness.
2. Prepare the avocado: Mash the avocado in a small bowl. Season with salt and pepper to taste.
3. Poach the egg: Fill a small saucepan with about 2 inches of water and bring to a simmer. Add the vinegar. Crack the egg into a small bowl. Swirl the water with a spoon to create a vortex. Gently slide the egg into the center of the vortex. Cook for 3-4 minutes, or until the whites are set and the yolk is cooked to your desired doneness. Remove the egg with a slotted spoon and drain on paper towels.
4. Assemble the toast: Spread the mashed avocado on the toasted bread. Top with the poached egg. Season with additional salt and pepper if desired.
5. Add optional toppings: Garnish with sliced cherry tomatoes, fresh herbs, or a drizzle of hot sauce, if desired.

Nutrition Information: Calories: 340, Fat: 17g, Protein: 12g, Fiber: 7g, Carbohydrates: 34g

Tips:

- Choose healthy fats like avocado, olive oil, and nuts instead of saturated and trans fats.
- Avoid processed foods and sugary drinks.
- Eat smaller, more frequent meals throughout the day instead of large, heavy meals.
- Drink plenty of water to stay hydrated.
- Talk to your doctor or a registered dietitian for personalized advice on managing your no-gallbladder diet.

Quinoa Breakfast Bowl

Cooking Time: 15 minutes | **Prep Time**: 10 minutes | **Total Time**: 25 minutes | **Serving Size**: 1

Ingredients:

- 1/2 cup quinoa, rinsed
- 1 cup water or low-fat broth
- 1/4 teaspoon ground cinnamon
- 1/4 teaspoon ground ginger
- 1/4 teaspoon ground turmeric
- Pinch of salt
- 1/4 cup berries (fresh or frozen)
- 1/4 banana, sliced
- 1/4 cup chopped nuts (walnuts, almonds, etc.)
- 1 tablespoon unsweetened yogurt or plant-based yogurt
- 1 tablespoon chia seeds
- Honey or maple syrup to taste (optional)

Directions:

1. Cook the quinoa: In a saucepan, combine quinoa, water or broth, spices, and salt. Bring to a boil, then reduce heat, cover, and simmer for 15 minutes, or until quinoa is fluffy and cooked through.
2. Prepare the toppings: While the quinoa cooks, wash and chop berries, slice banana, and chop nuts.
3. Assemble the bowl: Divide cooked quinoa evenly between two bowls. Top with berries, banana, nuts, yogurt, and chia seeds. Drizzle with honey or maple syrup, if desired.

Nutrition Information: Calories: 350, Fat: 8g, Saturated Fat: 2g, Cholesterol: 0mg, Carbohydrates: 45g, Fiber: 6g, Protein: 12g, Sodium: 200mg

Tips:

- Use any type of nut that you tolerate well. Pecans, cashews, and macadamia nuts are also good options.
- Add a dollop of mashed avocado for extra healthy fats and creaminess.
- If you prefer a warmer bowl, heat the berries before adding them.
- For a sweeter variation, substitute the plain yogurt with vanilla yogurt or add a touch of vanilla extract to the quinoa while cooking.
- Feel free to customize the toppings based on your preferences and dietary restrictions.

Cottage Cheese Pancakes

Prep Time: 5 minutes | **Cooking Time**: 10 minutes | **Total Time**: 15 minutes | **Servings**: 2

Ingredients:

- 1 cup small-curd cottage cheese
- 2 large eggs
- 1/4 cup all-purpose flour
- 1/2 teaspoon baking powder
- 1/4 teaspoon salt
- 1/4 teaspoon cinnamon (optional)
- 1 tablespoon milk (optional, if batter seems too thick)
- Cooking spray

Directions:

1. Combine wet ingredients: In a medium bowl, whisk together the cottage cheese and eggs until smooth.
2. Mix dry ingredients: In a separate bowl, whisk together the flour, baking powder, salt, and cinnamon (if using).
3. Combine wet and dry: Gradually add the dry ingredients to the wet ingredients, stirring until just combined. Do not over mix. The batter will be slightly thicker than traditional pancake batter.
4. Heat pan: Preheat a non-stick pan or griddle over medium heat. Spray with cooking spray.
5. Cook pancakes: Pour 1/4 cup of batter per pancake onto the hot pan. Cook for 2-3 minutes per side, or until golden brown and cooked through. If the batter seems too thick, you can add a tablespoon of milk to thin it slightly.
6. Serve: Serve immediately with your favorite toppings, such as fresh fruit, berries, or a drizzle of maple syrup.

Nutrition Information (per serving): Calories: 250, Fat: 6g, Saturated Fat: 2g, Cholesterol: 130mg, Protein: 20g, Carbohydrates: 25g, Fiber: 2g, Sugar: 5g

Tips:

- For a richer flavor, use full-fat cottage cheese.
- You can substitute gluten-free flour for a gluten-free option.
- Add a pinch of nutmeg or ginger to the batter for additional flavor.
- If you don't have a blender, you can mash the cottage cheese with a fork before adding it to the eggs.
- Make sure your pan is hot enough before adding the batter, otherwise the pancakes will stick.
- Don't overcook the pancakes, or they will become dry and tough.
- If you have any leftover batter, you can store it in the refrigerator for up to 24 hours.

Vegetable Frittata

Prep Time: 10 minutes | **Cooking Time**: 25 minutes | **Total Time**: 35 minutes | **Servings**: 4

Ingredients:

- 4 large eggs
- 1/4 cup low-fat milk or unsweetened almond milk
- 1/4 cup chopped red bell pepper
- 1/4 cup chopped green bell pepper
- 1/4 cup chopped zucchini
- 1/4 cup chopped mushrooms
- 1/4 cup chopped sun-dried tomatoes (oil-packed, drained)
- 1/4 cup chopped spinach
- 1/4 cup crumbled feta cheese (low-fat or fat-free option available)
- 1/4 cup shredded part-skim mozzarella cheese
- 1 tablespoon olive oil
- Salt and black pepper to taste

Directions:

1. Preheat oven to 375°F (190°C).
2. In a large bowl, whisk together eggs and milk until well combined. Season with salt and pepper.
3. Heat olive oil in an oven-safe skillet over medium heat. Add bell peppers, zucchini, and mushrooms. Cook for 5-7 minutes, until softened.
4. Stir in sun-dried tomatoes and spinach, cook for another minute until spinach wilts.
5. Pour egg mixture over the vegetables in the skillet. Top with feta and mozzarella cheese.
6. Bake for 20-25 minutes, or until the eggs are set and the center is no longer runny.
7. Let cool slightly before cutting into wedges and serving.

Nutrition Information: Calories: 250, Fat: 12g, Saturated Fat: 4g, Cholesterol: 210mg, Protein: 15g, Carbohydrates: 5g, Fiber: 2g, Sodium: 250mg

Tips:

- For a lighter option, use only egg whites instead of whole eggs.
- Add other vegetables suitable for the no gallbladder diet, like diced onion, chopped broccoli, or asparagus.
- Use herbs like basil, oregano, or thyme for extra flavor.
- Serve with a side of fruit or whole-wheat toast for a complete breakfast.

Chia Seed Pudding

Prep Time: 5 minutes | **Cooking Time**: None | **Total Time**: 10 minutes | **Serving** Size: 1

Ingredients:

- 1/4 cup chia seeds
- 1 cup unsweetened plant-based milk (almond, coconut, oat, etc.)
- 1 tablespoon maple syrup or other natural sweetener (optional)
- 1/2 teaspoon vanilla extract (optional)
- 1/4 teaspoon ground cinnamon (optional)
- Pinch of sea salt
- Toppings: Fresh fruit (berries, sliced banana, etc.), chopped nuts (almonds, walnuts, etc.), shredded coconut, unsweetened cocoa powder, nut butter (almond, peanut, etc.)

Directions:

1. In a small bowl or Mason jar, combine the chia seeds, milk, sweetener (if using), vanilla extract (if using), cinnamon, and salt. Stir well until everything is combined.
2. Cover the bowl or jar with a lid and refrigerate for at least 2 hours, or overnight for a thicker consistency.
3. In the morning, stir the pudding again to break up any clumps.
4. Top with your desired toppings and enjoy!

Nutrition Information: Calories: 230, Fat: 6g, Carbohydrates: 27g, Fiber: 11g, Protein: 5g

Tips:

- You can use any type of milk you like, but unsweetened plant-based milk is generally recommended for a no-gallbladder diet.
- If you prefer a sweeter pudding, you can add more maple syrup or another natural sweetener to taste.
- For a thicker pudding, use less milk or add more chia seeds.
- You can add other flavors to the pudding, such as cocoa powder, matcha powder, or spices like nutmeg or ginger.
- Chia pudding can be stored in the refrigerator for up to 3 days.

Banana Almond Butter Toast

Cooking Time: 5 minutes | **Prep Time**: 5 minutes | **Total Time**: 10 minutes | **Serving Size**: 1

Ingredients:

- 1 slice of whole-wheat bread
- 1 tablespoon of almond butter
- 1/2 banana, sliced
- ¼ teaspoon of ground cinnamon (optional)
- Sea salt to taste (optional)

Directions:

1. Toast the bread: Choose your preferred method, whether it's a toaster, pan-frying with a little olive oil, or broiling. Aim for a light golden brown toast.
2. Spread the almond butter: While the bread is warm, spread a generous tablespoon of almond butter evenly across the surface. Choose a creamy or crunchy variety as you prefer.
3. Top with banana slices: Arrange the banana slices evenly on top of the almond butter.
4. Season: Sprinkle with ground cinnamon for a warm and sweet flavor. A pinch of sea salt can also enhance the overall taste.
5. Enjoy! Serve immediately and savor the delicious and nutritious combination.

Nutrition Information: Calories: 250, Fat: 12g, Carbohydrates: 28g, Protein: 8g, Fiber: 3g, Potassium: 450mg

Tips:

- Choose whole-wheat bread: Opt for whole-wheat bread over white bread for added fiber and nutrients.
- Control the portion size: One slice of bread is ideal for the no gallbladder diet.
- Use low-fat nut butter: Look for almond butter labeled "low-fat" or "lite" to reduce the overall fat content.
- Substitute honey or maple syrup: If you find honey or maple syrup too rich, try sprinkling unsweetened shredded coconut for a touch of sweetness.
- Listen to your body: While this recipe is generally considered safe for the no gallbladder diet, always pay attention to how your body reacts and adjust accordingly.

Egg Muffins

Cooking Time: 20-25 minutes | **Prep Time**: 10 minutes | **Total Time**: 30-35 minutes |**Serving Size**: 6

Ingredients:

- 6 large eggs
- 1/2 cup chopped spinach
- 1/4 cup chopped bell pepper (any color)
- 1/4 cup chopped onion
- 1/4 cup crumbled feta cheese (low-fat option)
- 1/4 teaspoon dried oregano
- 1/4 teaspoon garlic powder
- Salt and pepper to taste
- Cooking spray

Directions:

1. Preheat oven to 375°F (190°C). Grease a muffin tin with cooking spray.
2. In a large bowl, whisk together the eggs.
3. Stir in the spinach, bell pepper, onion, feta cheese, oregano, garlic powder, salt, and pepper.
4. Divide the mixture evenly among the prepared muffin cups.
5. Bake for 20-25 minutes, or until the eggs are set and the centers are no longer runny.
6. Let cool slightly before serving.

   Nutrition Information: Calories: 150, Fat: 8g, Protein: 12g, Carbohydrates: 2g, Fiber: 1g

Tips:

- For added protein, stir in 1/4 cup cooked, lean chicken sausage or turkey bacon to the egg mixture.
- Add a dollop of low-fat Greek yogurt or mashed avocado to the top of each muffin for extra creaminess and healthy fats.
- Feel free to experiment with different vegetables and spices. Some other good options include chopped mushrooms, broccoli, or sun-dried tomatoes.
- Store leftover muffins in an airtight container in the refrigerator for up to 3 days. They can be reheated in the microwave or oven.

Yogurt and Fruit Smoothie

Cooking Time: None | **Prep Time**: 5 minutes | **Total Time**: 5 minutes | **Serving Size**: 1

Ingredients:

- 1 cup frozen fruit (choose low-fat options like berries, mango, pineapple, or papaya)
- 1/2 cup plain, low-fat Greek yogurt
- 1/4 cup unsweetened almond milk or oat milk
- 1/2 ripe banana (optional, for extra sweetness and creaminess)
- 1 tablespoon ground flaxseed (optional, for added fiber and omega-3s)
- 1/4 teaspoon ground cinnamon (optional, for flavor)
- Ice cubes, as needed

Directions:

1. Add all ingredients to a blender.
2. Blend until smooth and creamy, adding more ice cubes for a thicker consistency if desired.
3. Pour into a glass and enjoy!

Nutrition Information: Calories: 300-400, Fat: 4-8g, Protein: 15-20g, Carbohydrates: 30-40g, Fiber: 5-8g, Calcium: 300mg, Vitamin C: 50-100mg

Tips:

- Adjust the sweetness to your preference. You can use a natural sweetener like stevia or monk fruit instead of banana.
- Add a scoop of protein powder for an extra protein boost.
- Use dairy-free yogurt if you are lactose intolerant.
- Make sure all frozen fruits are suitable for the no-gallbladder diet. Avoid high-fat fruits like avocado and durian.
- This smoothie is a great base recipe. Feel free to experiment with different fruit combinations and add-ins like spinach, kale, or chia seeds.

Vegetable Omelette

Cooking Time: 15 minutes | **Prep Time**: 5 minutes | **Total Time**: 20 minutes | **Serving Size**: 1

Ingredients:

- 2 large eggs
- 1 tablespoon low-fat milk or unsweetened plant-based milk
- 1/4 teaspoon dried oregano
- Pinch of salt and black pepper
- 1 tablespoon olive oil
- 1/2 cup chopped bell pepper (any color)
- 1/4 cup chopped onion
- 1/4 cup chopped mushrooms
- 1/4 cup chopped spinach
- 1/4 cup shredded low-fat mozzarella cheese (optional)
- Chopped fresh herbs (optional, such as parsley, chives, or dill)

Directions:

1. Prep: Beat the eggs with milk, oregano, salt, and pepper in a small bowl. Chop the vegetables.
2. Cook vegetables: Heat olive oil in a non-stick frying pan over medium heat. Add onion and cook until softened, about 3 minutes. Add bell pepper and mushrooms and cook for another 2 minutes. Finally, add spinach and cook until wilted.
3. Cook omelette: Push the vegetables to one side of the pan. Pour in the egg mixture and let it cook for about 30 seconds, until the bottom starts to set. Tilt the pan to allow uncooked egg to flow towards the bottom.
4. Add fillings: Sprinkle mozzarella cheese over the omelette (if using) and top with the cooked vegetables.
5. Fold and finish: Fold the omelette in half and cook for another minute or two, until the cheese is melted and the eggs are cooked through.
6. Serve: Slide the omelette onto a plate and garnish with fresh herbs (if using). Enjoy immediately!

Nutrition Information: Calories: 250, Fat: 10g, Protein: 15g, Carbohydrates: 5g, Fiber: 2g

Tips:

- For added protein, you can add a crumbled cooked sausage patty or lean cooked ground turkey to the omelette.
- If you don't have mozzarella cheese, you can use another low-fat cheese or omit it altogether.
- Experiment with different vegetables based on your preferences and what you have on hand.
- Serve the omelette with a side of fruit or whole-wheat toast for a complete breakfast.

Buckwheat Pancakes

Prep Time: 10 minutes | **Cooking Time**: 15 minutes | **Total Time**: 25 minutes | **Serving Size**: 4

Ingredients:

- 1 cup buckwheat flour
- 1/2 cup all-purpose flour (optional, for a lighter texture)
- 1 tablespoon sugar
- 1 teaspoon baking powder
- 1/2 teaspoon baking soda
- 1/4 teaspoon salt
- 1 cup unsweetened almond milk
- 1 egg
- 1 tablespoon melted coconut oil
- 1 teaspoon vanilla extract

Directions:

1. In a large bowl, whisk together the buckwheat flour, all-purpose flour (if using), sugar, baking powder, baking soda, and salt.
2. In a separate bowl, whisk together the almond milk, egg, melted coconut oil, and vanilla extract.
3. Pour the wet ingredients into the dry ingredients and whisk just until combined. Do not over mix, as this can make the pancakes tough.
4. Heat a lightly greased griddle or skillet over medium heat. Pour 1/4 cup of batter onto the griddle for each pancake.
5. Cook for 2-3 minutes, or until bubbles appear on the surface of the pancakes. Flip the pancakes and cook for an additional 1-2 minutes, or until golden brown.
6. Serve immediately with your favorite no gallbladder diet toppings, such as fresh fruit, chopped nuts, or unsweetened applesauce.

Nutrition Information: Calories: 150, Fat: 4g, Saturated Fat: 1g Cholesterol: 0mg, Sodium: 200mg, Carbohydrates: 25g, Fiber: 3g, Sugar: 5g, Protein: 5g

Tips:

- For a richer flavor, use buttermilk instead of almond milk.
- You can add 1/4 cup of mashed ripe banana to the batter for added sweetness and moisture.
- If you don't have a griddle or skillet, you can make these pancakes on a regular pan.
- Leftover pancakes can be stored in the refrigerator for up to 3 days. Reheat them in a toaster or microwave before serving.

Salmon and Avocado Toast

Cooking Time: 5 minutes | **Prep Time**: 10 minutes | **Total Time**: 15 minutes | **Serving Size**: 1

Ingredients:

- 1 slice whole-wheat or gluten-free bread
- 1/2 ripe avocado
- 2 oz. poached salmon (see poaching instructions below)
- 1 tablespoon lemon juice
- 1/4 teaspoon dried dill
- Salt and pepper to taste
- Optional garnishes: chopped red onion, capers, fresh herbs (e.g., dill, chives)

Directions:

1. Poach the Salmon: Fill a small saucepan with 1-2 inches of water. Add a pinch of salt and a squeeze of lemon juice. Bring to a simmer. Gently slide the salmon fillet into the simmering water and cook for 4-5 minutes, or until just cooked through. Remove from the pan and flake with a fork.
2. Toast the Bread: While the salmon cooks, toast your bread to your desired level of doneness.
3. Prepare the Avocado: Mash the avocado in a small bowl with the lemon juice, dill, salt, and pepper.
4. Assemble the Toast: Spread the mashed avocado on the toasted bread. Top with the flaked salmon.
5. Garnish and Serve: Add your desired garnishes, such as chopped red onion, capers, or fresh herbs. Enjoy your delicious and nutritious breakfast!

Nutrition Information: Calories: 350, Fat: 18g, Carbohydrates: 25g, Protein: 20g, Fiber: 5g

Tips:

- For a richer flavor, add a drizzle of good-quality olive oil to the avocado mash.
- If you don't have fresh dill, you can substitute 1/8 teaspoon dried dill.
- Ensure the salmon is cooked through but not overcooked to avoid becoming tough.
- Use other low-fat protein options like poached chicken or shrimp if you prefer.
- Experiment with different toppings like sliced tomato, cucumber, or sprouts for added flavor and texture.

Fruit and Nut Breakfast Bowl

Cooking Time: 0 minutes | **Prep Time**: 5 minutes | **Total Time**: 5 minutes | **Serving Size**: 1 person

Ingredients

Base:
- 1/2 cup cooked rolled oats (cooked with water or unsweetened plant-based milk)
- 1/4 cup plain Greek yogurt (low-fat or fat-free)
- 1/4 cup unsweetened plant-based milk (optional, for desired consistency)

Toppings
- 1/2 cup fresh berries (blueberries, raspberries, strawberries)
- 1/4 cup chopped apple or pear
- 1/4 cup chopped banana
- 1 tablespoon chopped nuts (almonds, walnuts, pecans)
- 1 teaspoon chia seeds
- 1 teaspoon ground cinnamon (optional)
- Drizzle of honey or maple syrup (optional)

Directions:

1. Prepare the base: Cook the oats according to package instructions using water or unsweetened plant-based milk. Let cool slightly.
2. Assemble the bowl: In a bowl, combine the cooked oats, Greek yogurt, and plant-based milk (if using).
3. Add toppings: Top with your chosen fresh fruits, chopped nuts, chia seeds, and cinnamon.
4. Sweeten (optional): Drizzle with a small amount of honey or maple syrup if desired.

Nutrition Information: Calories: 300-400, Fat: 10-15g, Carbohydrates: 30-40g, Fiber: 5-10g, Protein: 5-10g

Tips:

- For a warm bowl, heat the cooked oats briefly in the microwave before assembling.
- Substitute different fruits based on your preference and seasonality.
- Use other low-fat dairy alternatives like kefir or unsweetened coconut yogurt.
- Add a scoop of protein powder for an extra protein boost.
- Sprinkle with shredded unsweetened coconut for added texture and flavor.
- Pre-chop fruits and nuts for even faster prep time.
- Feel free to adjust portion sizes based on your individual calorie needs.

Vegetable Breakfast Burrito

Prep Time: 10 minutes | **Cooking Time**: 15 minutes | **Total Time**: 25 minutes | **Servings**: 2

Ingredients:

- 2 large flour tortillas
- 2 large eggs, whites only (or 1/4 cup egg substitute)
- 1/2 red bell pepper, chopped
- 1/2 green bell pepper, chopped
- 1/2 cup chopped mushrooms
- 1/4 cup chopped onion
- 1/4 cup chopped spinach
- 1/4 cup shredded low-fat cheddar cheese
- 1/4 cup black beans, rinsed and drained
- 1/4 avocado, sliced (optional)
- Salt and pepper to taste
- Salsa or hot sauce (optional)

Directions:

1. Sauté the vegetables: Heat a large skillet over medium heat with a light coating of cooking spray. Add the bell peppers, mushrooms, and onion, and cook until softened, about 5 minutes. Add the spinach and cook until wilted.
2. Scramble the eggs: In a separate bowl, whisk the egg whites (or egg substitute) with salt and pepper. Pour into the skillet with the vegetables and scramble until cooked through.
3. Assemble the burritos: Warm the tortillas in a dry skillet or microwave for a few seconds. Spread each tortilla with a thin layer of cheese, then top with half of the egg mixture, black beans, and avocado (if using). Season with salt and pepper to taste.
4. Fold and roll: Fold the bottom of the tortilla up over the filling, then fold in the sides. Roll up tightly to enclose the filling.
5. Serve: Enjoy your burrito immediately, or wrap it in foil and store in the refrigerator for later. You can also toast the burrito in a dry skillet over medium heat for a few minutes before serving.

Nutrition Information: Calories: 350, Fat: 10g, Saturated Fat: 4g, Cholesterol: 200mg (if using egg yolks), Sodium: 300mg, Carbohydrates: 30g, Fiber: 5g, Protein: 15g

Tips:

- For a spicier burrito, add a pinch of red pepper flakes to the scrambled eggs.
- If you can tolerate a small amount of cholesterol, you can use whole eggs instead of just the whites.
- Feel free to add other vegetables to your liking, such as zucchini, broccoli, or cherry tomatoes.
- Serve your burrito with a side of fruit or yogurt for a complete breakfast.

Peanut Butter Banana Smoothie

Prep Time: 5 minutes | **Cooking Time**: 0 minutes | **Total Time**: 5 minutes | **Serving Size**: 1

Ingredients:

- 1 frozen banana
- 1/2 cup unsweetened almond milk (or other low-fat milk)
- 1 tablespoon creamy peanut butter (reduced-fat or natural)
- 1/2 cup plain Greek yogurt (low-fat or fat-free)
- 1/4 teaspoon ground cinnamon
- Optional: 1/2 scoop protein powder (unflavored or vanilla)
- Optional: 1 tablespoon chia seeds or flaxseed meal
- Optional: Handful of spinach or kale

Directions:

1. Add all ingredients to your blender in the order listed.
2. Blend until smooth and creamy, stopping to scrape down the sides as needed.
3. Adjust the consistency by adding more milk or ice cubes if desired.
4. Pour into a glass and enjoy immediately!

Nutrition Information: Calories: 350-400, Protein: 15-20g, Fat: 10-15g, Carbohydrates: 40-50g, Fiber: 5-10g, Sugar: 20-30g

Tips:

- Use frozen banana for a thicker smoothie.
- If you don't have a blender, you can use an immersion blender.
- For a creamier texture, add a ripe avocado.
- Boost the protein content with a scoop of protein powder.
- Add chia seeds or flaxseed meal for extra fiber and omega-3 fatty acids.
- For a green smoothie, add a handful of spinach or kale.
- For additional sweetness, use a small amount of natural sweetener like honey, maple syrup, or stevia.

Egg and Veggie Breakfast Casserole

Cooking Time: 40 minutes | **Prep Time**: 15 minutes | **Total Time**: 55 minutes | **Serving Size**: 8

Ingredients:

- 1 tablespoon olive oil
- 1/2 onion, diced
- 1 bell pepper, diced
- 1 cup chopped mushrooms
- 2 cups spinach, roughly chopped
- 1/2 cup crumbled low-fat feta cheese
- 8 large eggs
- 1/2 cup unsweetened almond milk
- 1/4 cup chopped fresh parsley
- 1/4 teaspoon dried thyme
- 1/4 teaspoon garlic powder
- Salt and pepper to taste

Directions:

1. Preheat oven to 375°F (190°C). Lightly grease a 9x13 inch baking dish.
2. Heat olive oil in a large skillet over medium heat. Add onion and bell pepper, and cook until softened, about 5 minutes. Add mushrooms and cook for another 3 minutes.
3. Stir in spinach and cook until wilted. Remove from heat and let cool slightly.
4. In a large bowl, whisk together eggs, almond milk, parsley, thyme, garlic powder, salt, and pepper.
5. Stir in cooled vegetables and feta cheese.
6. Pour mixture into prepared baking dish.
7. Bake for 40-45 minutes, or until eggs are set and casserole is golden brown.
8. Let cool slightly before serving.

Nutrition Information: Calories: 250, Protein: 15g, Fat: 10g, Fiber: 3g, Cholesterol: 200mg

Tips:

- For an extra flavor boost, add a pinch of red pepper flakes to the egg mixture.
- You can use any type of low-fat cheese that you like, such as mozzarella or Swiss.
- If you don't have fresh herbs, you can use 1/2 teaspoon dried parsley or thyme instead.
- To make this casserole ahead of time, prepare it as directed and then store it in the refrigerator overnight. Bake in the morning before serving.
- This casserole is also great for freezing. Let it cool completely, then wrap it tightly in foil and freeze for up to 3 months. Thaw overnight in the refrigerator before reheating.

Grilled Lemon Herb Chicken Salad

Cooking Time: 15 minutes | **Prep Time**: 10 minutes | **Total Time**: 25 minutes | **Serving Size**: 2 servings

Ingredients:

For the Chicken:
- 2 boneless, skinless chicken breasts (about 6 oz each)
- 1 tablespoon olive oil
- 1 tablespoon lemon juice
- 1/2 teaspoon dried oregano
- 1/4 teaspoon dried thyme
- 1/4 teaspoon garlic powder
- Salt and pepper to taste

For the Salad:
- 4 cups mixed greens (such as romaine, spinach, or baby kale)
- 1/2 cucumber, diced
- 1/2 red onion, thinly sliced
- 1/2 bell pepper, diced
- 1/4 cup cherry tomatoes, halved
- 1/4 cup crumbled feta cheese (optional)

For the Dressing:
- 2 tablespoons olive oil
- 1 tablespoon lemon juice
- 1/2 teaspoon Dijon mustard
- 1/4 teaspoon dried oregano
- 1/4 teaspoon dried thyme
- Salt and pepper to taste

Directions:
1. Marinate the chicken: In a bowl, whisk together olive oil, lemon juice, oregano, thyme, garlic powder, salt, and pepper. Add the chicken breasts and coat them evenly in the marinade. Cover and refrigerate for at least 30 minutes, or up to overnight for deeper flavor.
2. Prepare the salad: Wash and dry the greens. Dice the cucumber, red onion, and bell pepper. Halve the cherry tomatoes. Crumble the feta cheese (if using). Set aside.
3. Cook the chicken: Preheat a grill or grill pan to medium-high heat. Grill the chicken breasts for 5-7 minutes per side, or until cooked through and golden brown. Let cool slightly, then slice or shred the chicken.
4. Make the dressing: In a small bowl, whisk together olive oil, lemon juice, Dijon mustard, oregano, thyme, salt, and pepper.
5. Assemble the salad: Divide the greens between two plates. Top with the diced vegetables, sliced or shredded chicken, and crumbled feta cheese (if using). Drizzle with the dressing and serve immediately.

Nutrition Information: Calories: 350, Fat: 10g, Saturated Fat: 2g, Cholesterol: 60mg, Carbohydrates: 15g, Fiber: 3g, Protein: 35g

Tips:
- To make this salad ahead of time, prepare the chicken and salad ingredients earlier in the day. Store them separately in the refrigerator until ready to assemble.
- If you don't have a grill, you can bake the chicken in a preheated oven at 400°F for 15-20 minutes, or until cooked through.
- For a richer flavor, use grilled chicken thighs instead of breasts. However, keep in mind that thighs contain more fat and cholesterol.
- Feel free to experiment with different herbs and spices in the marinade and dressing.
- If you have dietary restrictions, be sure to choose ingredients that are appropriate for your needs.

Quinoa and Vegetable Stir-Fry

Cooking time: 20 minutes | **Prep time**: 10 minutes | **Total time**: 30 minutes | **Servings**: 2

Ingredients:

- 1 cup uncooked quinoa, rinsed
- 1 tablespoon olive oil
- 1 small onion, diced
- 1 clove garlic, minced
- 1 cup broccoli florets
- 1 cup bell pepper, sliced (any color)
- 1/2 cup snap peas, trimmed
- 1/4 cup cooked, shredded chicken breast (optional)
- 1/4 cup low-sodium soy sauce
- 1 tablespoon rice vinegar
- 1 teaspoon sesame oil
- 1/2 teaspoon cornstarch mixed with 1 tablespoon water
- Salt and pepper to taste
- Garnishes (optional): toasted sesame seeds, chopped green onions

Directions:

1. Cook the quinoa: Rinse the quinoa in a fine-mesh sieve. Combine the rinsed quinoa with 1 1/2 cups water in a saucepan. Bring to a boil, then reduce heat, cover, and simmer for 15 minutes or until fluffy. Remove from heat and fluff with a fork. Set aside.
2. Prepare the vegetables: While the quinoa cooks, dice the onion, mince the garlic, and chop the broccoli florets, bell pepper, and snap peas.
3. Cook the vegetables: Heat olive oil in a large skillet or wok over medium-high heat. Add the onion and cook for 2-3 minutes, until softened. Add the garlic and cook for another minute, until fragrant.
4. Stir-fry the vegetables: Add the broccoli, bell pepper, and snap peas to the skillet. Cook for 5-7 minutes, stirring occasionally, until the vegetables are tender-crisp.
5. Combine the ingredients: Add the cooked quinoa and optional chicken to the skillet. Stir to combine.
6. Make the sauce: In a small bowl, whisk together soy sauce, rice vinegar, sesame oil, and cornstarch mixture. Pour the sauce into the skillet and stir to coat everything evenly.
7. Season and serve: Season with salt and pepper to taste. Cook for another minute or two, until the sauce thickens slightly. Garnish with toasted sesame seeds and chopped green onions, if desired.

Nutrition information: Calories: 350, Fat: 5g, Saturated fat: 1g, Cholesterol: 0mg, Carbohydrates: 45g, Fiber: 5g, Protein: 15g

Tips:

- Use a variety of your favorite low-fat vegetables in this stir-fry. Some other good options include carrots, mushrooms, zucchini, or cabbage.
- If you don't have cooked chicken, you can omit it or substitute with tofu or tempeh.
- To make this stir-fry vegan, use vegetable broth instead of chicken broth in the sauce.
- Serve this stir-fry over brown rice or another whole grain for a more complete meal.
- If you have leftovers, store them in an airtight container in the refrigerator for up to 3 days.

Salmon and Avocado Wrap

Cooking Time: 10 minutes | **Prep Time**: 5 minutes | **Total Time**: 15 minutes | **Serving Size**: 1

Ingredients:

- 1 whole wheat tortilla
- 4 oz. skinless, boneless salmon fillet
- 1/2 avocado, sliced
- 1/4 cup chopped romaine lettuce
- 1/4 cup chopped cucumber
- 1 tablespoon plain Greek yogurt
- 1 tablespoon lemon juice
- 1/2 teaspoon Dijon mustard
- 1/4 teaspoon dried dill
- Pinch of salt and pepper

Directions:

1. Cook the salmon: You can bake, pan-fry, or grill the salmon to your preference. Here are two options:
2. Baking: Preheat oven to 400°F (200°C). Season the salmon with salt and pepper. Place on a baking sheet lined with parchment paper and bake for 10-12 minutes, or until cooked through.
3. Pan-frying: Heat a non-stick pan over medium heat with a drizzle of olive oil. Season the salmon with salt and pepper and cook for 3-4 minutes per side, or until cooked through.
4. While the salmon cooks, prepare the other ingredients:
5. Mash the avocado in a bowl with the lemon juice.
6. Combine the Greek yogurt, Dijon mustard, dill, salt, and pepper in a separate bowl.
7. Wash and chop the romaine lettuce and cucumber.
8. Assemble the wrap: Spread the Greek yogurt mixture onto the tortilla. Top with romaine lettuce, cucumber, avocado, and cooked salmon.
9. Roll up the wrap tightly and enjoy!

Nutrition Information: Calories: 350, Fat: 15g (3g saturated), Protein: 20g, Carbohydrates: 20g (5g fiber), Sodium: 200mg

Tips:
- For a spicier wrap, add a pinch of red pepper flakes to the yogurt mixture.
- If you don't have fresh dill, you can use 1/4 teaspoon dried dill.
- You can also add other vegetables to the wrap, such as shredded carrots, red onion, or bell peppers.
- Make sure to choose a whole wheat tortilla that is low in saturated fat and sodium.
- If you have any concerns about following a no gallbladder diet, it's always best to consult with a registered dietitian or healthcare professional.

Turkey and Hummus Veggie Wrap

Prep Time: 10 minutes | **Cooking Time:** 0 minutes | **Total Time:** 10 minutes **Servings:** 1

Ingredients:

- 1 whole wheat tortilla (spinach or whole wheat lavish are gallbladder-friendly options)
- 2 tablespoons hummus (choose a low-fat version if desired)
- 2-3 ounces sliced cooked turkey breast (grilled, roasted, or deli)
- 1/2 cup chopped romaine lettuce or spinach
- 1/4 cup shredded carrots
- 1/4 cup sliced cucumber
- 1/4 cup chopped red bell pepper
- 2 tablespoons crumbled feta cheese (optional)
- Fresh herbs (dill, parsley, mint) for garnish (optional)

Directions:

1. Spread the hummus evenly over half of the tortilla.
2. Layer the lettuce, carrots, cucumber, and bell pepper on top of the hummus.
3. Add the sliced turkey breast.
4. Fold the bottom half of the tortilla over the fillings, then fold the sides in to create a tight wrap.
5. Sprinkle with feta cheese and herbs, if desired.
6. Enjoy immediately!

Nutrition Information: Calories: 350, Fat: 10g, Saturated Fat: 3g, Cholesterol: 50mg, Sodium: 300mg, Carbohydrates: 30g, Fiber: 4g, Protein: 25g

Tips

- Choose lean cuts of turkey with minimal visible fat.
- Opt for low-fat or fat-free hummus.
- Limit cheese intake due to its fat content.
- Use fresh, raw vegetables instead of pickled or marinated options, which can be higher in sodium.
- Avoid spicy ingredients, which can irritate the digestive system.
- If you experience any discomfort after eating this wrap, adjust the ingredients or consult a healthcare professional for personalized dietary advice.

Mediterranean Chickpea Salad

Prep Time: 15 minutes | **Cooking Time**: None | **Total Time**: 15 minutes | **Servings**: 1

Ingredients:

- 1 cup cooked chickpeas, drained and rinsed
- 1/2 cucumber, diced
- 1/2 red bell pepper, diced
- 1/4 cup cherry tomatoes, halved
- 1/4 cup red onion, thinly sliced
- 2 tablespoons crumbled feta cheese (optional)
- 1 tablespoon chopped fresh parsley
- 2 tablespoons olive oil
- 1 tablespoon lemon juice
- 1/2 teaspoon dried oregano
- 1/4 teaspoon garlic powder
- Pinch of salt and black pepper

Directions:

1. Combine Salad Ingredients: In a large bowl, combine the chickpeas, cucumber, bell pepper, tomatoes, red onion, and feta cheese (if using).
2. Make the Dressing: In a small bowl, whisk together the olive oil, lemon juice, oregano, garlic powder, salt, and pepper.
3. Dress the Salad: Pour the dressing over the salad ingredients and toss gently to coat everything evenly.
4. Garnish and Serve: Sprinkle with fresh parsley and serve immediately.

Nutrition Information: Calories: 350, Fat: 10g, Saturated Fat: 2g, Cholesterol: 0mg, Carbohydrates: 40g, Fiber: 10g, Protein: 15g

Tips:

- For a creamier texture: Mash ¼ cup of the chickpeas with a fork before adding them to the salad.
- Customize the vegetables: Feel free to add other chopped vegetables like celery, olives, or artichoke hearts.
- Make it vegan: Omit the feta cheese and use a dairy-free vinaigrette.
- Storage: Leftovers can be stored in an airtight container in the refrigerator for up to 2 days. However, the salad texture might change slightly due to the tomatoes releasing more moisture.

Mediterranean Chickpea Salad

Prep Time: 15 minutes | **Cooking Time**: 0 minutes | **Total Time**: 15 minutes | **Servings**: 2

Ingredients:

- 1 (15oz) can chickpeas, drained and rinsed
- 1/2 cucumber, diced
- 1/2 red bell pepper, diced
- 1/4 cup red onion, finely diced
- 1/4 cup kalamata olives, pitted and halved
- 1/4 cup crumbled feta cheese (optional)
- 1/4 cup chopped fresh parsley
- 2 tablespoons olive oil
- 1 tablespoon lemon juice
- 1/2 teaspoon dried oregano
- 1/4 teaspoon garlic powder
- Salt and pepper to taste

Directions:

1. Combine the chickpeas, cucumber, bell pepper, red onion, olives, and parsley in a large bowl.
2. In a separate small bowl, whisk together the olive oil, lemon juice, oregano, garlic powder, salt, and pepper.
3. Pour the dressing over the chickpea mixture and toss to combine.
4. Taste and adjust seasonings as needed.
5. Serve immediately, or chill for at least 30 minutes for the flavors to develop.

Nutrition Information: Calories: 300, Fat: 6g, Saturated Fat: 1g, Cholesterol: 0mg, Sodium: 300mg, Carbohydrates: 35g, Fiber: 8g, Protein: 15g

Tips:

- For a creamier texture, mash some of the chickpeas with a fork before adding them to the salad.
- If you don't have fresh herbs, you can use 1 teaspoon dried oregano and 1/2 teaspoon dried parsley.
- This salad is also delicious served on a bed of lettuce or whole-wheat pita bread.
- To make this salad ahead of time, prepare all the ingredients but keep the dressing and salad separate until ready to serve.
- If you are new to the No Gallbladder Diet, it is best to start with a small portion of this salad and see how your body tolerates it.

Vegetable and Lentil Soup

Cooking Time: 30 minutes | **Prep Time**: 10 minutes | **Total Time**: 40 minutes | **Serving Size**: 4

Ingredients:

- 1 tablespoon olive oil
- 1 onion, chopped
- 2 carrots, chopped
- 2 celery stalks, chopped
- 2 cloves garlic, minced
- 1 cup brown lentils, rinsed
- 4 cups low-sodium vegetable broth
- 1 (14.5oz) can diced tomatoes, undrained
- 1 teaspoon dried oregano
- 1/2 teaspoon dried thyme
- Salt and pepper to taste
- Chopped fresh parsley, for garnish (optional)

Directions:

1. Heat olive oil in a large pot over medium heat. Add onion, carrots, and celery and cook for 5 minutes, until softened.
2. Add garlic and cook for an additional minute, until fragrant.
3. Add lentils, vegetable broth, tomatoes, oregano, and thyme. Bring to a boil, then reduce heat and simmer for 20 minutes, or until lentils are tender.
4. Season with salt and pepper to taste.
5. Serve hot, garnished with fresh parsley (optional).

Nutrition Information: Calories: 250, Fat: 4g, Carbohydrates: 35g, Fiber: 12g, Protein: 18g

Tips:

- For a smoother soup, remove half of the cooked lentils and puree them with a hand blender or immersion blender before returning them to the pot.
- You can substitute brown rice or quinoa for the lentils if desired.
- Add other vegetables to the soup, such as green beans, spinach, or chopped zucchini.
- Serve with a side of whole-wheat bread or crackers for a complete meal.

Tuna and White Bean Salad

Prep time: 10 minutes | **Cooking time**: 0 minutes | **Total time**: 10 minutes | **Servings**: 2

Ingredients:

- 1 (15-ounce) can tuna, packed in water, drained and flaked
- 1 (15-ounce) can white beans, rinsed and drained
- 1/2 cup chopped celery
- 1/4 cup chopped red onion
- 2 tablespoons chopped fresh parsley
- 2 tablespoons olive oil
- 1 tablespoon lemon juice
- 1/2 teaspoon dried dill
- Salt and pepper to taste

Directions:

1. In a large bowl, combine the tuna, white beans, celery, red onion, and parsley.
2. In a small bowl, whisk together the olive oil, lemon juice, dill, salt, and pepper.
3. Pour the dressing over the salad and toss to coat.
4. Serve immediately or refrigerate for up to 2 hours.

Nutrition information: Calories: 300, Fat: 10g, Saturated fat: 2g, Cholesterol: 30mg, Sodium: 400mg, Carbohydrates: 20g, Fiber: 5g, Sugar: 2g, Protein: 25g

Tips:

- For a creamier salad, mash some of the white beans with a fork before adding them to the salad.
- Add other chopped vegetables, such as cucumber or bell pepper, to the salad for more flavor and nutrients.
- If you don't have fresh herbs, you can use 1/2 teaspoon of dried dill or parsley.
- Serve the salad on a bed of lettuce or spinach for a more filling meal.

Grilled Veggie and Chicken Kabobs

Cooking Time: 15-20 minutes | **Prep Time**: 15 minutes | **Total Time**: 30-35 minutes | **Serving Size**: 2

Ingredients:

- 1 boneless, skinless chicken breast, cut into 1-inch pieces
- 1 medium zucchini, halved and cut into 1-inch pieces
- 1 red bell pepper, seeded and cut into 1-inch pieces
- 1/2 red onion, cut into 1-inch wedges
- 8 cherry tomatoes
- 2 tablespoons olive oil
- 1 tablespoon lemon juice
- 1/2 teaspoon dried oregano
- 1/4 teaspoon garlic powder
- 1/4 teaspoon salt
- 1/4 teaspoon black pepper
- Wooden skewers (soaked in water for 30 minutes)

Directions:

1. In a large bowl, whisk together olive oil, lemon juice, oregano, garlic powder, salt, and pepper. Add chicken pieces and coat evenly. Marinate for at least 30 minutes, or up to 2 hours.
2. Preheat grill to medium-high heat.
3. Thread chicken, zucchini, bell pepper, red onion, and cherry tomatoes onto skewers, alternating ingredients for even cooking.
4. Brush kabobs with remaining marinade.
5. Place kabobs on the grill and cook for 5-7 minutes per side, or until chicken is cooked through and vegetables are tender-crisp.
6. Serve immediately with your favorite dipping sauce, such as yogurt-based tzatziki or a vinaigrette.

Nutrition Information: Calories: 300, Fat: 10g, Carbs: 15g, Fiber: 3g, Protein: 30g

Tips:

- Use lean cuts of chicken, such as thighs or breasts.
- For a smoky flavor, add a few wood chips to the grill when preheating.
- If you don't have a grill, you can cook the kabobs in a grill pan or under the broiler.
- Make sure to cook the chicken until it is cooked through to an internal temperature of 165°F (74°C).
- Be careful not to overcook the vegetables, as they will become mushy.
- Feel free to experiment with different vegetables, such as mushrooms, asparagus, or pineapple.
- For added protein, you can also add shrimp or tofu to the kabobs.

Shrimp and Avocado Salad

Cooking Time: 5 minutes | **Prep Time**: 10 minutes | **Total Time**: 15 minutes | **Serving Size**: 1

Ingredients:

- 1/2 pound raw shrimp, peeled and deveined
- 1 ripe avocado, pitted and diced
- 1/2 cucumber, diced
- 1/4 red onion, diced
- 1/4 cup cherry tomatoes, halved
- 1/4 cup chopped fresh cilantro
- 2 tablespoons olive oil
- 1 tablespoon lemon juice
- 1/2 teaspoon dried oregano
- 1/4 teaspoon garlic powder
- Salt and black pepper to taste

Directions:

1. Cook the shrimp: Bring a pot of water to a boil. Add the shrimp and cook for 2-3 minutes, or until pink and cooked through. Drain and cool.
2. Assemble the salad: In a large bowl, combine the avocado, cucumber, red onion, tomatoes, cilantro, and cooked shrimp.
3. Make the dressing: In a small bowl, whisk together the olive oil, lemon juice, oregano, garlic powder, salt, and pepper.
4. Dress the salad: Pour the dressing over the salad and toss to coat. Serve immediately.

Nutrition Information: Calories: 350, Fat: 15g, Carbohydrates: 10g, Protein: 25g, Fiber: 3g, Cholesterol: 150mg, Sodium: 300mg

Tips:

- For a spicier salad, add a pinch of red pepper flakes to the dressing.
- If you don't have fresh cilantro, you can substitute parsley or another fresh herb.
- To make this salad ahead of time, cook the shrimp and store it in the refrigerator. Assemble the salad just before serving.
- Be mindful of portion sizes, especially when it comes to shrimp and avocado, as they are higher in calories.
- Adjust the seasoning to your taste.
- Consider using low-sodium ingredients to keep the sodium content in check.

Vegetable and Turkey Sauté

Cooking Time: 20 minutes | **Prep Time**: 10 minutes | **Total Time**: 30 minutes | Serving Size: 2

Ingredients:

- 1 tablespoon olive oil
- 1/2 onion, chopped
- 1 clove garlic, minced
- 1 cup ground turkey
- 1 cup bell peppers (assorted colors), chopped
- 1 cup broccoli florets
- 1/2 cup cherry tomatoes, halved
- 1/4 cup chicken broth
- 1/2 teaspoon dried oregano
- 1/4 teaspoon black pepper
- Salt to taste
- 1/4 cup chopped fresh parsley (optional)

Directions:

1. Prep: Wash and chop all vegetables. Preheat a large skillet over medium heat.
2. Sauté aromatics: Heat olive oil in the skillet. Add onion and cook for 3-4 minutes until softened. Add garlic and cook for another minute, stirring constantly.
3. Cook the turkey: Add ground turkey to the pan and break it up with a spoon. Cook for 5-7 minutes until browned and cooked through.
4. Add vegetables: Add bell peppers, broccoli, and cherry tomatoes to the pan. Stir fry for 3-4 minutes until vegetables are slightly softened but still crisp-tender.
5. Simmer and flavor: Pour in chicken broth, oregano, black pepper, and salt. Bring to a simmer and cook for 2-3 minutes, allowing the flavors to meld.
6. Serve: Garnish with fresh parsley (optional) and serve hot with brown rice, quinoa, or whole-wheat pasta.

Nutrition Information: Calories: 350, Fat: 10g, Saturated Fat: 3g, Cholesterol: 50mg, Protein: 35g, Carbohydrates: 20g, Fiber: 5g

Tips:

- For a spicier flavor, add a pinch of red pepper flakes with the garlic.
- You can substitute ground turkey with cooked chicken breast or lean ground beef.
- Feel free to add other low-fat vegetables like zucchini, asparagus, or mushrooms.
- If you have leftover cooked turkey, you can use it instead of cooking raw ground turkey.

DINNER RECIPES

Grilled Lemon Herb Chicken with Steamed Vegetables

Cooking Time: 25 minutes | **Prep Time**: 10 minutes | **Total Time**: 35 minutes | **Serving Size**: 2

Ingredients:

For the chicken:
- 2 boneless, skinless chicken breasts (150g each)
- 1 tablespoon olive oil
- 1 tablespoon lemon juice
- 1 teaspoon dried oregano
- 1/2 teaspoon dried thyme
- 1/4 teaspoon garlic powder
- Salt and pepper to taste

For the vegetables:
- 1 cup broccoli florets
- 1 cup baby carrots
- 1/2 cup green beans
- 1/4 cup water

Directions:

1. Marinate the chicken: In a small bowl, whisk together the olive oil, lemon juice, oregano, thyme, garlic powder, salt, and pepper. Place the chicken breasts in a shallow dish and pour the marinade over them, coating them evenly. Let the chicken marinate for at least 30 minutes, or up to 2 hours.
2. Prepare the steamer: Fill a pot with about 1 inch of water and bring it to a boil. Place a steamer basket in the pot and make sure it sits above the water without touching it.
3. Steam the vegetables: Add the broccoli, carrots, and green beans to the steamer basket. Cover the pot and steam the vegetables for 5-7 minutes, or until tender-crisp.
4. Grill the chicken: Preheat your grill to medium-high heat. Grill the chicken breasts for 6-8 minutes per side, or until cooked through. An instant-read thermometer inserted into the thickest part of the chicken should reach 165°F (74°C).
5. Serve: Serve the grilled chicken with the steamed vegetables and enjoy!

Nutrition Information: Calories: 350, Fat: 10g, Protein: 40g, Carbohydrates: 15g, Fiber: 3g per

Tips:

- You can use any type of fresh or dried herbs that you like in the marinade.
- If you don't have a grill, you can bake the chicken in a preheated oven at 400°F (200°C) for 20-25 minutes, or until cooked through.
- Serve the chicken and vegetables with a drizzle of olive oil and a squeeze of fresh lemon juice.
- For added flavor, you can grill some lemon slices alongside the chicken.

Turkey and Vegetable Stir-Fry

Prep Time: 15 minutes | **Cooking Time**: 15 minutes | **Total Time**: 30 minutes | **Servings**: 4

Ingredients:

- 1 tablespoon olive oil
- 1/2 pound ground turkey breast
- 1 onion, diced
- 2 bell peppers (different colors), sliced
- 1 cup broccoli florets
- 1 cup snap peas, trimmed
- 1 carrot, julienned
- 1 clove garlic, minced (optional)
- 1/2 teaspoon ginger, grated (optional)
- 1/4 cup low-sodium soy sauce
- 2 tablespoons chicken broth
- 1 tablespoon cornstarch
- 1/4 cup chopped fresh cilantro
- 1/4 cup cooked brown rice (optional, for serving)

Directions:

1. Prep the vegetables: Wash and chop all vegetables according to the instructions above. Set aside.
2. Cook the turkey: Heat olive oil in a large skillet or wok over medium-high heat. Add the ground turkey and cook until browned, breaking it up with a spoon as it cooks.
3. Add vegetables and aromatics: Once the turkey is cooked, add the onion, bell peppers, and broccoli. Sauté for 5 minutes, then add the snap peas and carrot. Stir-fry for another 3 minutes, or until the vegetables are slightly softened but still crisp-tender.
4. Make the sauce: In a small bowl, whisk together soy sauce, chicken broth, and cornstarch. Pour the sauce into the skillet with the vegetables and stir to combine.
5. Finish the stir-fry: If using, add the garlic and ginger and cook for another 30 seconds. Stir in the chopped cilantro and cook for an additional minute.
6. Serve: Serve the stir-fry over cooked brown rice, if desired.

Nutrition Information per Serving: Calories: 250, Fat: 5g, Saturated Fat: 1g, Cholesterol: 50mg, Carbohydrates: 20g, Fiber: 5g Protein: 30g

Tips:

- For a thicker sauce, mix the cornstarch with a tablespoon of water before adding it to the sauce mixture.
- Feel free to add other vegetables that are suitable for the no-gallbladder diet, such as zucchini, mushrooms, or snow peas.
- If you don't have ground turkey, you can use lean chicken breast, shredded.
- To make the recipe egg-free, skip adding the egg white or use a cornstarch slurry instead.
- Serve with a side of cooked quinoa or whole-wheat noodles for a more complete meal.

Baked Cod with Lemon Garlic Butter Sauce and Steamed Green Beans

Prep Time: 10 minutes | **Cooking Time**: 15-20 minutes | **Total Time**: 25-30 minutes | **Servings**: 2

Ingredients:

- 2 cod fillets (4-6 oz each), skinless and boneless
- 1 tablespoon olive oil
- 2 tablespoons lemon juice
- 2 cloves garlic, minced
- ¼ teaspoon dried thyme
- Salt and pepper to taste
- ½ cup fresh green beans, trimmed
- 2 tablespoons water
- Fresh parsley, chopped (optional)

Directions:

1. Preheat oven to 400°F (200°C). Lightly grease a baking dish.
2. In a small bowl, whisk together olive oil, lemon juice, garlic, thyme, salt, and pepper.
3. Place cod fillets in the prepared baking dish. Pour the lemon-garlic sauce over the cod, ensuring it is evenly coated.
4. In a separate microwave-safe dish, combine green beans and water. Cover and microwave on high for 2-3 minutes, or until beans are tender-crisp. Drain any excess water.
5. Bake the cod for 15-20 minutes, or until it is opaque and flakes easily with a fork.
6. While the cod bakes, arrange the steamed green beans alongside the fish in the baking dish.
7. Broil the fish for an additional 1-2 minutes, if desired, for a slightly browned top.
8. Garnish with chopped fresh parsley, if using. Serve immediately.

Nutrition Information (per serving): Calories: 250, Fat: 10g, Saturated Fat: 2g, Cholesterol: 50mg, Sodium: 150mg, Carbohydrates: 5g, Fiber: 2g, Protein: 30g

Tips:

- Use low-fat or fat-free butter or yogurt instead of regular butter in the sauce for a lower-fat option.
- Experiment with other herbs and spices, such as oregano, basil, or paprika, to add different flavors.
- Serve with quinoa, brown rice, or roasted vegetables for a complete and balanced meal.
- Adjust the cooking time based on the thickness of your cod fillets.

Shrimp and Veggie Skewers with Brown Rice

Cooking Time: 20 minutes | **Prep Time**: 15 minutes | **Total Time**: 35 minutes | **Servings**: 4

Ingredients:

- 1 pound large shrimp, peeled and deveined (remove any veins for gallbladder sensitivity)
- 1 tablespoon olive oil
- 1/2 teaspoon paprika
- 1/4 teaspoon garlic powder
- 1/4 teaspoon onion powder
- 1/4 teaspoon black pepper
- 1 bell pepper, cut into 1-inch chunks
- 1 zucchini, cut into 1-inch chunks
- 1 red onion, cut into 1-inch wedges
- 1 cup cooked brown rice
- 1/4 cup chopped fresh parsley, for garnish (optional)

Directions:

1. Marinate the shrimp: In a bowl, combine olive oil, paprika, garlic powder, onion powder, and black pepper. Add shrimp and toss to coat evenly. Marinate for at least 15 minutes, or up to 30 minutes.
2. Prepare the vegetables: Preheat oven to 400°F (200°C). Thread bell pepper, zucchini, and onion onto skewers, alternating vegetables for variety.
3. Cook the skewers: Place skewers on a baking sheet lined with parchment paper. Bake for 10-12 minutes, or until shrimp are cooked through and vegetables are tender.
4. Warm the brown rice: While the skewers bake, warm the brown rice in a microwave or saucepan according to package instructions.
5. Assemble and serve: Divide brown rice among plates. Top with cooked shrimp and veggie skewers. Garnish with fresh parsley, if desired.

Nutrition Information: Calories: 350, Fat: 10g, Saturated Fat: 2g, Cholesterol: 200mg, Sodium: 300mg, Carbohydrates: 30g, Fiber: 5g, Protein: 25g

Tips:

- For a smokier flavor, grill the skewers on an outdoor grill instead of baking them.
- Substitute other low-fat protein options like skinless chicken breast or tofu if desired.
- Experiment with different vegetables like cherry tomatoes, mushrooms, or broccoli.
- Serve with a low-fat dipping sauce like lemon juice, yogurt, or salsa.
- Make sure to remove any visible veins from the shrimp, as these can be difficult to digest and trigger gallbladder discomfort.
- Adjust the seasoning to your preference, but be mindful of sodium intake if you have other dietary

Baked Salmon with Quinoa and Roasted Asparagus

Cooking Time: 25 minutes | **Prep Time**: 10 minutes | **Total Time**: 35 minutes |**Serving Size**: 2

Ingredients:

- 2 (6-oz) skinless salmon fillets
- 1 tablespoon olive oil
- 1/2 teaspoon dried thyme
- 1/4 teaspoon garlic powder
- Salt and black pepper, to taste
- 1 cup quinoa, rinsed
- 1 1/2 cups water or vegetable broth
- 1 bunch asparagus, trimmed
- 1 tablespoon lemon juice
- 1/4 cup chopped fresh parsley (optional)

Directions:

1. Preheat oven to 400°F (200°C) Line a baking sheet with parchment paper.
2. Prepare the salmon: In a small bowl, combine olive oil, thyme, garlic powder, salt, and pepper. Rub the mixture onto both sides of the salmon fillets.
3. Cook the quinoa: In a medium saucepan, combine quinoa and water or broth. Bring to a boil, then reduce heat, cover, and simmer for 15 minutes, or until fluffy and all liquid is absorbed. Fluff with a fork.
4. Roast the asparagus: While the quinoa cooks, toss asparagus with a drizzle of olive oil and sprinkle with salt and pepper. Arrange on one half of the prepared baking sheet.
5. Bake the salmon: Place the salmon fillets on the other half of the baking sheet. Bake for 15-20 minutes, or until the salmon is cooked through and flakes easily with a fork.
6. Assemble and serve: Divide the quinoa among two plates. Top with roasted asparagus and a salmon fillet. Drizzle with lemon juice and sprinkle with fresh parsley, if desired.

Nutrition Information: Calories: 450, Protein: 35g, Fat: 15g, Carbohydrates: 40g, Fiber: 5g, Sodium: 300mg

Tips:

- For added flavor, you can marinate the salmon in your favorite marinade for 30 minutes before baking.
- Substitute brown rice for quinoa if desired.
- Experiment with different herbs and spices to customize the flavor of the dish.
- If you have concerns about sodium intake, omit the salt or use a low-sodium alternative.
- For a richer flavor, consider using low-fat Greek yogurt instead of lemon juice.

Vegetarian Chili with Whole Grain Bread

Prep Time: 15 minutes | **Cook Time**: 30 minutes | **Total Time**: 45 minutes || **Servings**: 4

Ingredients:

- 1 tablespoon olive oil
- 1 medium onion, chopped
- 2 cloves garlic, minced
- 1 green bell pepper, chopped
- 1 red bell pepper, chopped
- 1 jalapeno pepper, seeded and chopped (optional)
- 1 teaspoon ground cumin
- 1 teaspoon chili powder
- ½ teaspoon smoked paprika
- ¼ teaspoon cayenne pepper (optional)
- 1 (15-ounce) can diced tomatoes, undrained
- 1 (14.5-ounce) can diced fire-roasted tomatoes, undrained
- 1 (15-ounce) can black beans, rinsed and drained
- 1 (15-ounce) can pinto beans, rinsed and drained
- 1 (14.5-ounce) can vegetable broth
- 1 bay leaf
- Salt and pepper to taste
- 4 slices whole-wheat bread, toasted
- Optional toppings: chopped avocado, chopped cilantro, lime wedges, low-fat cheese

Directions:

1. Heat olive oil in a large pot or Dutch oven over medium heat. Add onion and cook until softened, about 5 minutes. Stir in garlic, bell peppers, and jalapeno (if using) and cook for 2-3 minutes more, until softened.
2. Add cumin, chili powder, paprika, and cayenne pepper (if using) and cook for 1 minute, stirring constantly, to toast the spices.
3. Add diced tomatoes, fire-roasted tomatoes, black beans, pinto beans, vegetable broth, and bay leaf. Bring to a boil, then reduce heat to low and simmer for 20 minutes, stirring occasionally.
4. Season with salt and pepper to taste. Remove bay leaf before serving.
5. To serve, ladle chili onto toasted whole-wheat bread slices. Add desired toppings, such as chopped avocado, cilantro, lime wedges, or low-fat cheese.

Nutrition Information: Calories: 350, Fat: 8g, Saturated Fat: 2g, Cholesterol: 0mg, Carbohydrates: 50g, Fiber: 12g, Protein: 15g

Tips:

- For a thicker chili, mash some of the beans with a fork before adding them to the pot.
- You can adjust the spice level to your preference.
- Feel free to add other vegetables to the chili, such as corn, zucchini, or carrots.
- Serve with a side salad for a complete meal.

Tofu Stir-Fry with Brown Rice

Cooking Time: 20 minutes | **Prep Time**: 10 minutes | **Total Time**: 30 minutes | **Serving Size**: 2

Ingredients:
- 1 cup cooked brown rice
- 1 block (14oz) firm tofu, drained and pressed
- 1 tablespoon olive oil
- 1/2 onion, diced
- 2 cloves garlic, minced
- 1 cup broccoli florets
- 1 cup bell pepper (any color), sliced
- 1/2 cup carrots, julienned
- 1/4 cup snow peas
- 1/4 cup low-sodium soy sauce
- 1 tablespoon rice vinegar
- 1 tablespoon cornstarch mixed with 2 tablespoons water
- 1/4 teaspoon ginger powder
- Pinch of black pepper
- Optional toppings: sesame seeds, chopped green onions, sriracha

Directions:
1. Cook the brown rice: If you haven't already, cook the brown rice according to package instructions. Set aside.
2. Prepare the tofu: Cut the tofu into cubes or slices. It's important to drain and press the tofu well to remove excess moisture.
3. Heat the oil: Heat the olive oil in a large wok or skillet over medium-high heat.
4. Sauté the onions and garlic: Add the onions and garlic to the pan and cook until softened, about 3 minutes.
5. Stir-fry the vegetables: Add the broccoli, bell pepper, and carrots to the pan and cook for 5 minutes, stirring occasionally.
6. Add the snow peas and tofu: Add the snow peas and tofu to the pan and cook for another 2-3 minutes, until the tofu is golden brown and the vegetables are tender-crisp.
7. Make the sauce: In a small bowl, whisk together the soy sauce, rice vinegar, cornstarch mixture, ginger powder, and black pepper.
8. Thicken the sauce: Pour the sauce into the pan with the vegetables and tofu. Stir constantly until the sauce thickens and coats the ingredients.
9. Serve: Serve the stir-fry over cooked brown rice. Garnish with optional toppings, such as sesame seeds, chopped green onions, or sriracha.

Nutrition Information per Serving: Calories: 400, Fat: 10g, Cholesterol: 0mg, Sodium: 300mg, Carbohydrates: 50g, Fiber: 5g, Protein: 20g

Tips:
- You can use any type of vegetables you like in this stir-fry. Just make sure they are gallbladder-friendly, such as broccoli, bell peppers, carrots, snow peas, mushrooms, and leafy greens.
- If you don't have cornstarch, you can use arrowroot powder or tapioca starch instead.
- To make the sauce even lower in sodium, use low-sodium soy sauce or tamari.
- Serve with a side of steamed chicken or fish for a more complete meal.
- If you are sensitive to soy, you can use tamari or coconut aminos instead of soy sauce.

Grilled Chicken Caesar Salad

Prep Time: 15 minutes | **Cooking Time**: 20 minutes | **Total Time**: 35 minutes | **Servings**: 2

Ingredients:

For the chicken:
- 2 boneless, skinless chicken breasts
- 1 tablespoon olive oil
- 1/2 teaspoon dried oregano
- 1/4 teaspoon garlic powder
- 1/4 teaspoon onion powder
- Salt and black pepper to taste

For the salad:
- 2 romaine hearts, chopped
- 1/2 cup cherry tomatoes, halved
- 1/4 cup red onion, thinly sliced
- 1/4 cup shaved Parmesan cheese
- 2 tablespoons reduced-fat Caesar salad dressing (check for gallbladder-friendly options)
- Optional: 1/4 cup homemade croutons (recipe below)

For the croutons (optional):
- 1 slice whole-wheat bread, cubed
- 1 tablespoon olive oil
- 1/4 teaspoon garlic powder
- Pinch of salt

Directions:

1. Marinate the chicken: In a bowl, combine olive oil, oregano, garlic powder, onion powder, salt, and pepper. Add chicken breasts and coat evenly. Marinate for at least 15 minutes, or up to 30 minutes for more flavor.
2. Prepare the croutons (optional): Preheat oven to 375°F (190°C). Toss bread cubes with olive oil, garlic powder, and salt. Spread on a baking sheet and bake for 5-7 minutes, or until golden brown and crispy.
3. Cook the chicken: Heat a grill pan over medium heat. Grill chicken breasts for 5-7 minutes per side, or until cooked through. Alternatively, bake chicken in a preheated oven at 400°F (200°C) for 15-20 minutes, or until internal temperature reaches 165°F (74°C).
4. Assemble the salad: In a large bowl, combine romaine lettuce, tomatoes, red onion, and Parmesan cheese.
5. Slice the chicken: Once cooked, let the chicken rest for a few minutes before slicing it into thin strips.
6. Dress the salad: Drizzle the reduced-fat Caesar salad dressing over the salad and toss to coat. Add the sliced chicken and croutons (if using).
7. Serve immediately and enjoy

Nutrition Information: Calories: 350 per serving, Fat: 15g, Saturated Fat: 4g, Cholesterol: 70mg, Sodium: 450mg, Carbohydrates: 10g, Fiber: 2g, Protein: 40g

Tips:

- For a more flavorful marinade, add a tablespoon of lemon juice or balsamic vinegar.
- If you don't have a grill pan, you can cook the chicken in a skillet over medium heat.
- To make the salad even more filling, add cooked quinoa or brown rice.
- If you can't tolerate store-bought Caesar dressing, try making your own with olive oil, lemon juice, Dijon mustard, Parmesan cheese, and seasonings.
- Be sure to check the ingredients in all packaged products to ensure they are suitable for a No Gallbladder Diet.

Quinoa Stuffed Bell Peppers

Cooking Time: 45 minutes | **Prep Time**: 15 minutes | **Total Time**: 60 minutes | **Servings**: 4

Ingredients:

- 4 large bell peppers (red, yellow, orange, or a mix)
- 1 cup uncooked quinoa, rinsed
- 1 1/2 cups vegetable broth
- 1 tablespoon olive oil
- 1 medium onion, chopped
- 2 cloves garlic, minced
- 1/2 cup diced celery
- 1 (15 oz) can diced tomatoes, drained
- 1 (15 oz) can black beans, rinsed and drained
- 1/2 cup frozen corn
- 1/4 cup chopped fresh cilantro
- 2 tablespoons nutritional yeast (optional)
- 1/2 teaspoon ground cumin
- 1/4 teaspoon paprika
- Salt and pepper to taste

Directions:

1. Preheat oven to 375°F (190°C) Line a baking dish with parchment paper.
2. Prepare the bell peppers: Wash and halve the bell peppers lengthwise, removing the seeds and membranes.
3. Cook the quinoa: Rinse the quinoa thoroughly. In a saucepan, combine the quinoa and vegetable broth. Bring to a boil, then reduce heat, cover, and simmer for 15 minutes or until the quinoa is cooked and fluffy. Fluff with a fork and set aside.
4. Sauté the vegetables: Heat olive oil in a large skillet over medium heat. Add the onion, celery, and garlic, and sauté until softened, about 5 minutes.
5. Combine the filling: Add the diced tomatoes, black beans, corn, cooked quinoa, cilantro, nutritional yeast (if using), cumin, paprika, salt, and pepper to the skillet. Stir to combine and cook for an additional 5 minutes.
6. Stuff the peppers: Divide the filling evenly among the prepared bell peppers. Place the stuffed peppers upright in the baking dish.
7. Bake: Bake for 30-35 minutes, or until the peppers are tender and the filling is heated through.
8. Serve: Enjoy hot, garnished with additional fresh cilantro (optional).

Nutrition Information: Calories: 350, Fat: 8g, Protein: 15g, Fiber: 8g, Carbohydrates: 35g, Sodium: 300mg

Tips:
- For a spicier kick, add a chopped jalapeno to the sautéed vegetables.
- Use brown rice instead of quinoa for a different texture.
- If you don't have vegetable broth, use low-sodium chicken broth or water.
- Top with your favorite low-fat cheese, such as feta or crumbled goat cheese, before baking for an extra layer of flavor (optional).
- Leftovers can be stored in an airtight container in the refrigerator for up to 3 days.

Vegetable and Chickpea Curry with Cauliflower Rice

Cooking Time: 25 minutes | **Prep Time**: 15 minutes | **Total Time**: 40 minutes | **Servings**: 4

Ingredients:

- 1 tablespoon olive oil
- 1 medium onion, diced
- 2 cloves garlic, minced
- 1 inch ginger, grated
- 1 teaspoon ground turmeric
- 1 teaspoon ground cumin
- 1/2 teaspoon coriander powder
- 1/4 teaspoon chili powder (optional)
- 1 (14.5oz) can diced tomatoes, undrained
- 1 (13.5oz) can light coconut milk
- 1 cup vegetable broth
- 1 cup frozen peas
- 1 cup chopped broccoli florets
- 1 (15oz) can chickpeas, drained and rinsed
- 1/2 cup chopped fresh cilantro
- Salt and pepper to taste

For the Cauliflower Rice:

- 1 head cauliflower, cut into florets

Directions:

1. Prepare the cauliflower rice: Pulse the cauliflower florets in a food processor until rice-like consistency is achieved. You can also grate the cauliflower using the large holes of a box grater. Set aside.
2. Heat the oil in a large pot or Dutch oven over medium heat. Add the onion and cook until softened, about 5 minutes. Add the garlic and ginger, cook for another minute, stirring frequently.
3. Stir in the turmeric, cumin, coriander, and chili powder (if using). Cook for 30 seconds, allowing the spices to bloom.
4. Add the diced tomatoes, coconut milk, vegetable broth, peas, and broccoli. Bring to a simmer and cook for 10 minutes, until the vegetables are tender.
5. Stir in the chickpeas and cauliflower rice. Season with salt and pepper to taste. Simmer for an additional 5 minutes, or until the cauliflower rice is cooked through.
6. Remove from heat and stir in the cilantro. Serve immediately.

Nutrition Information: Calories: 350, Fat: 8g, Carbohydrates: 30g, Fiber: 8g, Protein: 15g

Tips:

- For a creamier curry, use full-fat coconut milk.
- If you don't have a food processor, you can grate the cauliflower using the large holes of a box grater.
- You can add other vegetables to this curry, such as carrots, bell peppers, or zucchini.
- Serve this curry with a side of brown rice or quinoa for a complete meal.
- Adjust the spices to your preference.

Greek yogurt with berries

Cooking Time: 0 minutes | **Prep Time**: 5 minutes | **Total Time**: 5 minutes | **Serving Size**: 1 person

Ingredients:

- 1 cup plain Greek yogurt
- 1/2 cup fresh berries (such as blueberries, raspberries, strawberries, or blackberries)
- 1/4 cup chopped nuts (optional)
- 1 tablespoon honey (or maple syrup) (optional)
- 1/2 teaspoon ground cinnamon (optional)

Directions:

1. In a bowl, combine the Greek yogurt, berries, nuts (if using), honey (if using), and cinnamon (if using).
2. Stir gently to combine all ingredients.
3. Enjoy immediately!

Nutrition Information: Calories: 200, Fat: 2g, Saturated Fat: 1g, Cholesterol: 5mg, Sodium: 80mg, Carbohydrates: 20g, Fiber: 4g, Sugar: 15g, Protein: 15g

Tips:

- For a thicker yogurt, use strained Greek yogurt.
- You can use any type of berries that you like.
- If you are looking for a sweeter snack, you can add more honey or maple syrup.
- For a more protein-packed snack, add a scoop of protein powder to the yogurt.
- This recipe is easily doubled or tripled to make a larger serving.

Hummus with sliced vegetables

Cooking Time: 10 minutes | **Prep Time**: 10 minutes | **Total Time**: 20 minutes | **Serving Size**: 4

Ingredients:

- 1 can (15 oz) chickpeas, drained and rinsed (or 1 cup dried chickpeas, cooked and cooled)
- 2 tablespoons tahini
- 2 tablespoons olive oil
- 1/4 cup lemon juice
- 2 cloves garlic, minced
- 1/2 teaspoon ground cumin
- 1/4 teaspoon salt
- Black pepper to taste
- Assorted sliced vegetables, such as carrots, cucumbers, bell peppers, celery, and radishes (choose low-fat options like cucumbers and radishes)

Directions:

1. Make the hummus: If using dried chickpeas, cook them according to package instructions. Drain and rinse well.
2. In a food processor, combine the chickpeas, tahini, olive oil, lemon juice, garlic, cumin, salt, and pepper. Blend until smooth and creamy, scraping down the sides as needed. Taste and adjust seasonings as desired.
3. Prepare the vegetables: Wash and slice the vegetables into bite-sized pieces.
4. Assemble the snack: Arrange the sliced vegetables on a plate and serve with the hummus. Enjoy!

Nutrition Information: Calories: 200g, Fat: 5g, Saturated Fat: 1g, Cholesterol: 0mg, Protein: 7g, Fiber: 5g, Carbohydrates: 20g, Sodium: 200mg

Tips:

- For a smoother hummus, remove the skins from the chickpeas before blending. You can do this by rubbing the cooked chickpeas between your fingers after rinsing them.
- If you don't have tahini, you can substitute peanut butter or another nut butter.
- Add a sprinkle of paprika or cayenne pepper to the hummus for a bit of heat.
- Serve the hummus with whole-wheat pita bread or crackers for a more filling snack.
- This recipe is easily doubled or tripled to make a larger batch.

Apple slices with almond butter

Prep Time: 5 minutes | **Cooking Time**: 0 minutes | **Total Time**: 5 minutes | **Serving Size**: 1

Ingredients:

- 1 medium apple (tart varieties like Granny Smith work well)
- 2 tablespoons almond butter (smooth or crunchy, depending on preference)
- Optional toppings: cinnamon, raisins, unsweetened shredded coconut, chopped nuts (avoid high-fat nuts like pecans)

Directions:

1. Wash and prepare the apple: Thoroughly wash the apple and remove the core using an apple corer or knife.
2. Slice the apple: Cut the apple into thin slices or bite-sized chunks.
3. Spread the almond butter: Spread a thin layer of almond butter onto each apple slice or chunk. Use a knife or spoon for even distribution.
4. Add toppings (optional): If desired, sprinkle with a pinch of cinnamon, raisins, unsweetened shredded coconut, or chopped nuts. Choose healthy, low-fat nut options like almonds or cashews.
5. Enjoy! Serve immediately and savor the delicious and nutritious snack.

Nutrition Information: Calories: 180, Fat: 13g, Protein: 3g, Carbohydrates: 21g, Sugar: 16g, Sodium: 2mg

Tips:

- For variety, try different apple varieties like Honey crisp, Fuji, or Gala.
- Use homemade almond butter for more control over ingredients and reduced sodium.
- Drizzle a small amount of honey or maple syrup for an extra touch of sweetness, but remember it will increase the sugar content.
- Enjoy this snack as part of a balanced diet rich in fruits, vegetables, and whole grains.
- Consult your doctor or a registered dietitian for personalized dietary guidance specific to your gallbladder health.

Cottage cheese with pineapple

Cooking Time: 0 minutes | **Prep Time**: 5 minutes | **Total Time**: 5 minutes | **Serving Size**: 1

Ingredients:

- 1/2 cup (125g) low-fat cottage cheese
- 1/4 cup (60g) fresh pineapple, chopped
- 1 tablespoon chopped walnuts or pecans (optional)
- 1/4 teaspoon ground cinnamon (optional)
- Fresh mint leaves, for garnish (optional)

Directions:

1. In a small bowl, combine the cottage cheese and pineapple.
2. Stir in the walnuts or pecans, if using.
3. Sprinkle with cinnamon, if using.
4. Garnish with fresh mint leaves, if desired.

Nutrition Information: Calories: 160, Protein: 14g, Carbohydrates: 18g, Fat: 3g, Fiber: 2g, Sugar: 14g

Tips:

- For a sweeter snack, use canned pineapple in its own juice. Drain the juice before adding the pineapple to the cottage cheese.
- You can substitute other fruits for the pineapple, such as mango, papaya, or berries.
- Add a drizzle of honey or maple syrup for additional sweetness.
- If you have a blender, you can blend the ingredients together for a smoother consistency.
- This recipe is easily doubled or tripled to make a larger serving.

Edamame

Cooking Time: 5 minutes | **Prep Time**: 5 minutes | **Total Time**: 10 minutes |**Serving Size**: 1

Ingredients:

- 1 cup frozen shelled edamame
- 1/2 teaspoon olive oil
- 1/4 teaspoon sea salt (optional)
- Spices of your choice (e.g., garlic powder, black pepper, chili flakes, paprika)

Directions:

1. Thaw the edamame: If using frozen edamame, thaw it in the microwave according to package instructions or by placing it in a colander under cold running water for 5 minutes.
2. Heat the olive oil: In a large skillet or saucepan, heat the olive oil over medium heat.
3. Add the edamame: Once the oil is hot, add the thawed edamame and cook for 3-4 minutes, stirring occasionally, until heated through.
4. Seasoning: Sprinkle with salt (if desired) and you're chosen spices. Toss to coat evenly.
5. Serve immediately: Enjoy your edamame warm as a satisfying and healthy snack.

Nutrition Information: Calories: 180, Fat: 9g, Protein: 17g, Carbohydrates: 13g, Fiber: 8g, Sodium: 180mg

Tips:

- For a richer flavor, use toasted sesame oil instead of olive oil.
- Add a squeeze of fresh lemon juice for a zesty twist.
- Consider adding other low-fat ingredients like chopped fresh herbs, roasted garlic, or a sprinkle of nutritional yeast.
- Be mindful of portion sizes, as even healthy snacks can contribute to excess calorie intake.

Trail mix

Cooking Time: None | **Prep Time**: 10 minutes | **Total Time**: 10 minutes | **Serving Size**: 1/4

Ingredients:

Sweet Mix

- 1/4 cup dry roasted almonds
- 1/4 cup dry roasted cashews
- 1/4 cup pumpkin seeds
- 1/4 cup dried cranberries
- 1/4 cup dried cherries (unsweetened)
- 1/4 cup raisins (optional)

Savory Mix:

- 1/4 cup dry roasted chickpeas
- 1/4 cup dry roasted pepitas (pumpkin seeds)
- 1/4 cup dry roasted sunflower seeds
- 1/4 cup whole-wheat pretzels (broken into bite-sized pieces)
- 1/4 cup dried cranberries (unsweetened)
- 1/4 cup dried apricots (unsweetened)

Optional Add-ins (for both mixes):

- Dried banana chips (unsweetened)
- Roasted seaweed snacks
- Air-popped popcorn (low-fat)
- Unsweetened shredded coconut flakes

Directions:

1. Prepare a clean, airtight container.
2. Measure out each ingredient according to your chosen mix or customize based on your preferences.
3. Combine all ingredients in the container.
4. Mix well and enjoy!

Nutrition Information (per serving): Calories: Around 200-250, Fat: Less than 10 grams, Saturated Fat: Less than 2 grams, Cholesterol: Minimal, Fiber: Around 5-7 grams, Sugar: Varies depending on the chosen dried fruit

Tips:

- Store your trail mix in an airtight container in a cool, dry place for up to a week.
- Adjust the quantities of each ingredient to your liking.
- Be mindful of portion sizes, as even healthy snacks can add up in calories.
- Consider the fat content of different nuts and seeds. Opt for low-fat options like almonds, cashews, and pumpkin seeds.
- Substitute ingredients as needed based on your dietary restrictions or preferences.

Grilled Vegetable Skewers

Cooking Time: 10-15 minutes | **Prep Time**: 15 minutes | **Total Time**: 25-30 minutes | **Serving Size**: 4

Ingredients:

- 1 zucchini, cut into 1-inch pieces
- 1 yellow squash, cut into 1-inch pieces
- 1 red bell pepper, cut into 1-inch pieces
- 1 green bell pepper, cut into 1-inch pieces
- 1 small onion, cut into 1-inch wedges
- 8 cherry tomatoes
- 1 tablespoon olive oil
- 1/2 teaspoon dried oregano
- 1/4 teaspoon garlic powder
- 1/4 teaspoon salt
- 1/4 teaspoon black pepper
- Wooden skewers (soaked in water for at least 30 minutes)

Directions:

1. Preheat grill to medium-high heat.
2. In a large bowl, combine zucchini, squash, bell peppers, onion, and cherry tomatoes.
3. In a small bowl, whisk together olive oil, oregano, garlic powder, salt, and pepper. Pour over vegetables and toss to coat evenly.
4. Thread vegetables onto soaked wooden skewers, alternating colors and types of vegetables for visual appeal.
5. Grill skewers for 5-7 minutes per side, or until vegetables are tender and slightly charred.
6. Serve immediately and enjoy!

Nutrition Information: Calories: 150, Fat: 5g, Saturated Fat: 1g, Cholesterol: 0mg, Carbohydrates: 15g, Fiber: 3g, Protein: 5g

Tips:

- For a smoky flavor, add a few wood chips to the grill when preheating.
- If you don't have a grill, you can broil the skewers in the oven for 10-12 minutes per side.
- Serve with a low-fat dipping sauce, such as a yogurt-based tzatziki or a light vinaigrette.
- Feel free to experiment with different vegetables, such as eggplant, mushrooms, or asparagus.
- Make sure to choose low-fat cooking methods, such as grilling or broiling, to avoid adding unhealthy fats to your diet.

Hummus with Veggie Sticks

Cooking Time: None | **Prep Time**: 10 minutes | **Total Time**: 10 minutes | **Serving Size**: 4-6

Ingredients:

- 1 (15-ounce) can no-fat or low-fat chickpeas, drained and rinsed
- 2 tablespoons tahini (sesame paste)
- 2 tablespoons lemon juice
- 1 clove garlic, minced
- 1/4 cup water
- 1/4 teaspoon ground cumin
- 1/8 teaspoon salt (or to taste)
- Black pepper to taste
- Assorted fresh vegetables, such as cucumber, carrots, celery, bell peppers, and broccoli florets (for dipping)

Directions:

1. In a food processor, combine the chickpeas, tahini, lemon juice, garlic, water, cumin, salt, and black pepper. Process until smooth and creamy, scraping down the sides as needed. Adjust seasonings to taste.
2. Transfer the hummus to a serving bowl. Garnish with a drizzle of olive oil and a sprinkle of paprika, if desired.
3. Arrange the veggie sticks around the hummus for dipping. Enjoy!

Nutrition Information: Calories: 170, Fat: 6g, Saturated Fat: 1g, Cholesterol: 0mg, Sodium: 280mg , Carbohydrates: 20g, Fiber: 5g, Protein: 7g

Tips:

- For a creamier hummus, add more water, 1 tablespoon at a time, until desired consistency is reached.
- If you don't have tahini, you can substitute peanut butter or another nut butter.
- Get creative with your veggie sticks! Try other options like cherry tomatoes, radishes, or jicama.
- To make this recipe even more no-gallbladder friendly, opt for low-sodium hummus and limit your sodium intake throughout the day.
- You can store leftover hummus in an airtight container in the refrigerator for up to 3 days.

Caprese Salad Skewers

Prep Time: 10 minutes | **Cooking Time**: None | **Total Time**: 10 minute | **Serving Size**: 10

Ingredients:

- 20 grape tomatoes (mixed colors optional)
- 10 ounces mozzarella cheese, cubed (low-fat or fat-free if preferred)
- 20 fresh basil leaves
- 2 tablespoons extra virgin olive oil (use sparingly if needed)
- 1/4 teaspoon dried oregano (optional)
- 1/4 teaspoon dried basil (optional)
- Salt and freshly ground black pepper to taste

Directions:

1. Wash and dry the tomatoes and basil leaves.
2. Cut the mozzarella cheese into cubes roughly the same size as the tomatoes.
3. If using, whisk together the olive oil, oregano, and dried basil in a small bowl.
4. Assemble the skewers: thread one tomato, one basil leaf, and one mozzarella cube onto each skewer. Repeat with remaining ingredients.
5. Drizzle lightly with the olive oil mixture if desired. Season with salt and pepper to taste.
6. Serve immediately.

Nutrition Information: Calories: 70, Fat: 5g, Saturated Fat: 3g, Cholesterol: 15mg, Sodium: 100mg, Carbohydrates: 4g, Fiber: 1g, Sugar: 2g, Protein: 4g

Tips:

- Limit fat: Opt for low-fat or fat-free mozzarella cheese. Use olive oil sparingly or consider omitting it altogether for a completely fat-free option.
- Choose wisely: Select ripe, flavorful tomatoes to compensate for reduced fat.
- Skip the extras: Avoid garnishes like fried capers or pesto, which can add unwanted fat.
- Listen to your body: Start with a small portion and adjust based on your individual tolerance.

Cucumber Roll-Ups

Cooking Time: 5 minutes | **Prep Time**: 10 minutes | **Total Time**: 15 minutes | **Serving Size**: 12 roll-ups

Ingredients:

- 1 medium cucumber, thinly sliced lengthwise
- 4 oz. reduced-fat cream cheese, softened
- 1/4 cup finely chopped fresh dill
- 1 tablespoon lemon juice
- 1/4 teaspoon salt
- 1/4 teaspoon black pepper
- Optional fillings: Chopped smoked salmon, crumbled cooked shrimp, finely chopped red bell pepper, or a sprinkle of everything bagel seasoning

Directions:

1. Make the cream cheese mixture: In a small bowl, combine the softened cream cheese, dill, lemon juice, salt, and pepper. Mix until well combined and smooth.
2. Prepare the cucumber slices: Lay the cucumber slices flat on a cutting board. If the slices are very wide, you can trim them slightly on the sides to make them easier to roll.
3. Assemble the roll-ups: Spread a thin layer of the cream cheese mixture on each cucumber slice. Add a sprinkle of your chosen filling (if using), then carefully roll up the cucumber slice from one end to the other.
4. Chill and serve: Refrigerate the roll-ups for at least 30 minutes before serving. This allows the flavors to meld and the cucumber to soften slightly.

Nutrition Information: Calories: 50, Fat: 3g, Carbohydrates: 5g, Fiber: 1g, Protein: 2g

Tips:

- Use a mandolin slicer for perfectly even and thin cucumber slices.
- If you don't have fresh dill, you can substitute 1/2 teaspoon dried dill.
- To make the roll-ups ahead of time, assemble them and store them in an airtight container in the refrigerator for up to 24 hours.
- For a richer flavor, use full-fat cream cheese. However, keep in mind that this will increase the fat content per serving.
- Get creative with your fillings! Experiment with different combinations of flavors and textures to find your favorites.

Stuffed Mushrooms

Prep Time: 15 minutes | **Cooking Time**: 20 minutes | **Total Time**: 35 minutes | **Serving Size**: 6-8

Ingredients:

- 8 large cremini mushrooms (cleaned and stems removed)
- 1 tablespoon olive oil
- 1/2 onion, finely chopped
- 1 clove garlic, minced
- 1/2 cup cooked, shredded chicken or turkey (**optional** for added protein)
- 1/4 cup low-fat ricotta cheese
- 1/4 cup chopped spinach
- 1/4 cup chopped fresh parsley
- 1/4 cup grated Parmesan cheese
- 1/4 teaspoon dried oregano
- Salt and pepper to taste

Directions:

1. Preheat oven to 375°F (190°C). Line a baking sheet with parchment paper.
2. In a large skillet, heat olive oil over medium heat. Add onion and cook until softened, about 5 minutes. Add garlic and cook for another minute, until fragrant.
3. Stir in cooked chicken or turkey (if using). Cook for 2-3 minutes, until heated through.
4. In a separate bowl, combine ricotta cheese, spinach, parsley, Parmesan cheese, oregano, salt, and pepper. Mix well.
5. Spoon the ricotta mixture into the prepared mushroom caps, filling them evenly.
6. Place the stuffed mushrooms on the prepared baking sheet. Bake for 20 minutes, or until the filling is golden brown and bubbly.
7. Let cool slightly before serving.

Nutrition Information: Calories: 100, Fat: 5g, Cholesterol: 0mg, Sodium: 300mg, Fiber: 2g, Protein: 5g

Tips:

- For a vegetarian option, replace the chicken or turkey with cooked lentils or quinoa.
- You can also use different types of mushrooms, such as Portobello or white button mushrooms.
- To make ahead, stuff the mushrooms and refrigerate for up to 24 hours before baking.
- Sprinkle with additional fresh herbs before serving for a pop of color and flavor.

Shrimp Cocktail

Cooking Time: 3 minutes | **Prep Time**: 10 minutes | **Total Time**: 13 minutes | **Serving Size**: 4

Ingredients:

- 1 pound large shrimp, peeled and deveined
- 4 cups water
- 1 tablespoon lemon juice
- 1/2 teaspoon salt
- 1/4 teaspoon black pepper
- 1/4 teaspoon ground cayenne pepper (optional)
- 1/2 cup cocktail sauce (low-fat or homemade)
- 1/4 cup chopped fresh parsley
- Lemon wedges, for garnish

Directions:

1. Poach the shrimp: In a large pot, bring the water, lemon juice, salt, pepper, and cayenne pepper (if using) to a boil. Add the shrimp and cook for 3 minutes, or until just pink and opaque. Remove from heat and drain, discarding the poaching liquid.
2. Chill the shrimp: Rinse the shrimp under cold water and transfer them to a bowl. Cover and refrigerate for at least 30 minutes, or until chilled through.
3. Assemble the cocktail: Divide the chilled shrimp among four serving glasses. Drizzle with cocktail sauce and sprinkle with parsley. Garnish with lemon wedges and serve immediately.

Nutrition Information: Calories: 120, Fat: 1g, Cholesterol: 170mg, Sodium: 300mg, Carbohydrates: 1g, Protein: 20g

Tips:

- For a milder flavor, omit the cayenne pepper.
- You can use frozen shrimp, thawed and patted dry, for this recipe.
- Make your own low-fat cocktail sauce by combining ketchup, horseradish, lemon juice, and spices to taste.
- Serve the shrimp cocktail with your favorite low-fat crackers or vegetables for a complete appetizer.

Guacamole with Baked Tortilla Chips

Cooking Time: 20 minutes | **Prep Time**: 10 minutes | **Total Time**: 30 minutes | **Serving Size**: 4

Ingredients:

For the Baked Tortilla Chips:

- 6 corn tortillas
- 1 tablespoon olive oil
- 1/2 teaspoon garlic powder
- 1/4 teaspoon smoked paprika
- 1/4 teaspoon salt

For the Guacamole:

- 2 ripe avocados, halved, pitted, and peeled
- 1/4 cup red onion, finely diced
- 1/4 cup roma tomato, finely diced
- 1/4 cup fresh cilantro, chopped
- 1 tablespoon lime juice
- 1/2 teaspoon ground cumin
- 1/4 teaspoon salt
- Pinch of black pepper

Directions:

For the Baked Tortilla Chips

1. Preheat oven to 375°F (190°C). Line a baking sheet with parchment paper.
2. Brush tortillas lightly with olive oil.
3. In a small bowl, combine garlic powder, paprika, and salt. Sprinkle the spice mixture evenly over the tortillas.
4. Cut tortillas into wedges or triangles. Arrange them in a single layer on the prepared baking sheet.
5. Bake for 15-20 minutes, or until golden brown and crispy, flipping halfway through.
6. Let cool slightly before serving.

For the Guacamole:

1. In a large bowl, mash the avocados with a fork or potato masher until desired consistency is reached. You can leave it chunky or smooth, depending on your preference.
2. Stir in the red onion, roma tomato, cilantro, lime juice, cumin, salt, and black pepper.
3. Taste and adjust seasonings as needed.

Nutrition Information: Calories: 200, Fat: 14g, Fiber: 5g, Carbohydrates: 15g, Protein: 4g

Tips:

- For a smoother guacamole, remove the skin from the avocados before mashing.
- If you don't have roma tomatoes, you can use another type of tomato, such as cherry tomatoes.
- Add a little jalapeño pepper for a spicy kick, but be sure to remove the seeds and pith first if you have a sensitive stomach.
- Serve the guacamole immediately to prevent browning. You can squeeze a little extra lime juice on top to help prevent browning as well.
- Store leftover guacamole in an airtight container in the refrigerator for up to 24 hours.

Quinoa Stuffed Peppers

Cooking Time: 35 minutes | **Prep Time**: 15 minutes | **Total Time**: 50 minutes | **Serving Size**: 4

Ingredients:

- 2 bell peppers (red, yellow, or orange), halved and seeds removed
- 1/2 cup quinoa, rinsed
- 1 cup vegetable broth
- 1 tablespoon olive oil
- 1/2 onion, diced
- 1 clove garlic, minced
- 1/2 cup chopped mushrooms
- 1/4 cup chopped cherry tomatoes
- 1/4 cup cooked black beans, rinsed and drained
- 1/4 cup chopped fresh cilantro
- 1/4 cup crumbled feta cheese (optional)
- Salt and pepper to taste

Directions:

1. Preheat oven to 375°F (190°C). Line a baking dish with parchment paper.
2. Cook the quinoa: In a saucepan, combine quinoa and vegetable broth. Bring to a boil, then reduce heat and simmer for 15 minutes, or until quinoa is cooked through and fluffed. Set aside.
3. Prepare the filling: While the quinoa cooks, heat olive oil in a large skillet over medium heat. Add onion and cook until softened, about 5 minutes. Add garlic and cook for an additional minute until fragrant.
4. Stir in mushrooms and cook until browned. Add cherry tomatoes and cook for another 2 minutes.
5. Add cooked quinoa, black beans, and cilantro to the skillet. Stir to combine and season with salt and pepper to taste.
6. Stuff the peppers: Divide the quinoa mixture evenly between the prepared bell peppers. Top with crumbled feta cheese (optional).
7. Bake for 20-25 minutes, or until peppers are tender and filling is heated through.
8. Let cool slightly before serving. Enjoy!

Nutrition Information: Calories: 250, Fat: 8g, Saturated Fat: 2g, Cholesterol: 0mg, Carbohydrates: 35g, Fiber: 6g, Protein: 10g

Tips:

- For a spicier version, add a pinch of red pepper flakes to the filling.
- You can substitute the feta cheese with another low-fat cheese like ricotta or mozzarella.
- If you don't have fresh cilantro, you can use 1 teaspoon of dried cilantro.
- Serve with a dollop of plain yogurt or a side salad for a complete meal.

Cucumber Tomato Salad Cups

Cooking Time: None | **Prep Time**: 15 minutes | **Total Time**: 15 minutes | **Serving Size**: 4

Ingredients:

- 2 large cucumbers, washed and peeled
- 2 medium tomatoes, cored and diced
- 1/4 cup red onion, finely diced (optional)
- 1/4 cup fresh herbs (such as parsley, dill, or chives), chopped
- 1 tablespoon lemon juice
- 1 tablespoon olive oil
- 1/4 teaspoon salt
- 1/4 teaspoon black pepper

Directions:

1. Prepare the cucumbers: Using a spiralizer or mandolin, cut the cucumbers into long, thin ribbons. Alternatively, you can use a vegetable peeler to create wide, thin strips.
2. Assemble the cups: Lay the cucumber ribbons flat on a plate, overlapping slightly to create a circle. Gently press the center down to form a cup shape. Repeat with remaining cucumber ribbons to create 4 cups.
3. Prepare the salad: In a bowl, combine diced tomatoes, red onion (if using), and fresh herbs.
4. Make the dressing: In a separate bowl, whisk together lemon juice, olive oil, salt, and pepper.
5. Fill the cups: Gently spoon the tomato mixture into each cucumber cup. Drizzle with the dressing and serve immediately.

Nutrition Information: Calories: 60, Fat: 1g, Cholesterol: 0mg, Carbohydrates: 10g, Fiber: 2g, Protein: 2g, Sodium: 130mg

Tips:

- For a creamier texture, substitute plain Greek yogurt for some of the olive oil in the dressing.
- Add a touch of sweetness with a pinch of honey or a drizzle of balsamic vinegar.
- If you don't have a spiralizer or mandolin, thinly slice the cucumbers with a knife.
- Make sure to remove the seeds from the tomatoes to avoid excess acidity, which can be irritating for a No Gallbladder Diet.
- Feel free to experiment with different herbs and spices to personalize the flavor.
- Serve this appetizer chilled for a refreshing start to your meal.

Chicken and Vegetable Soup

Cooking Time: 30 minutes | **Prep Time**: 15 minutes | **Total Time**: 45 minutes | **Serving Size**: 4

Ingredients

- 1 tablespoon olive oil
- 1 onion, diced
- 2 carrots, diced
- 2 celery stalks, diced
- 2 cloves garlic, minced
- 4 cups low-sodium chicken broth
- 1 pound boneless, skinless chicken breast, cubed
- 1 cup chopped green beans
- 1 cup chopped broccoli florets
- 1/2 cup frozen peas
- 1/4 cup chopped fresh parsley
- Salt and pepper to taste

Directions:

1. Heat olive oil in a large pot or Dutch oven over medium heat. Add onion, carrots, and celery and cook until softened, about 5 minutes.
2. Add garlic and cook for an additional minute until fragrant.
3. Pour in chicken broth and bring to a boil.
4. Reduce heat to simmer and add chicken breast cubes. Cook for 10-15 minutes, or until chicken is cooked through and opaque.
5. Add green beans, broccoli, and peas to the pot. Simmer for an additional 5-7 minutes, or until vegetables are tender-crisp.
6. Stir in fresh parsley and season with salt and pepper to taste.
7. Serve immediately and enjoy!

Nutrition Information: Calories: 220, Fat: 5g, Saturated Fat: 1g, Cholesterol: 60mg, Sodium: 500mg, Carbohydrates: 15g, Fiber: 3g, Protein: 25g

Tips:

- For a thicker soup, remove some of the cooked vegetables and mash them with a fork before returning them to the pot.
- You can use other low-fat vegetables in this soup, such as zucchini, spinach, or mushrooms.
- If you are sensitive to sodium, use low-sodium chicken broth or vegetable broth.
- To make the soup ahead of time, let it cool completely and store in the refrigerator for up to 3 days. Reheat gently before serving.

Butternut Squash Soup

Cooking Time: 30 minutes | **Prep Time**: 10 minutes | **Total Time**: 40 minutes | **Serving Size**: 4

Ingredients:

- 1 medium butternut squash, peeled and cubed
- 1 medium onion, chopped
- 2 cloves garlic, minced
- 1 tablespoon olive oil
- 4 cups vegetable broth
- 1 teaspoon ground ginger
- 1/2 teaspoon ground cinnamon
- 1/4 teaspoon ground nutmeg
- Salt and pepper to taste
- Chopped fresh parsley, for garnish (optional)

Directions:

1. In a large pot, heat olive oil over medium heat. Add onion and cook until softened, about 5 minutes.
2. Add garlic and cook for an additional minute, until fragrant.
3. Add butternut squash, vegetable broth, ginger, cinnamon, and nutmeg. Bring to a boil, then reduce heat and simmer for 20-25 minutes, or until squash is tender.
4. Let soup cool slightly, then puree in batches in a blender or food processor until smooth.
5. Return soup to pot and season with salt and pepper to taste.
6. Serve hot, garnished with fresh parsley (optional).

Nutrition Information: Calories: 180, Fat: 5g, Cholesterol: 0mg, Sodium: 300mg, Carbohydrates: 25g, Fiber: 5g, Protein: 4g

Tips:

- For a richer flavor, you can roast the butternut squash before adding it to the soup. Simply toss the cubed squash with olive oil and salt, then roast in a preheated oven at 400°F for 20-25 minutes, or until tender.
- If you don't have vegetable broth, you can use chicken broth or water. However, chicken broth will add more fat and sodium to the soup.
- You can also add other vegetables to this soup, such as carrots, celery, or potatoes.
- To make the soup vegan, omit the garnish of parsley.

Turkey Chili

Prep Time: 15 minutes | **Cooking Time**: 30 minutes | **Total Time**: 45 minutes | **Serving Size**: 4-6

Ingredients:

- 1 tablespoon olive oil
- 1 medium onion, chopped
- 2 cloves garlic, minced
- 1 green bell pepper, chopped
- 1 pound ground turkey (93% lean or higher)
- 1 (28-ounce) can crushed tomatoes, no salt added
- 1 (15-ounce) can black beans, rinsed and drained
- 1 (15-ounce) can pinto beans, rinsed and drained
- 1 (14.5-ounce) can diced tomatoes, no salt added
- 1 tablespoon chili powder
- 1 teaspoon ground cumin
- 1/2 teaspoon smoked paprika
- 1/4 teaspoon cayenne pepper (optional, for a kick)
- 1/4 teaspoon black pepper
- 1/2 cup low-sodium chicken broth
- 1 tablespoon cornstarch (optional, for thickening)
- Chopped fresh cilantro, for garnish (optional)

Directions:

1. Heat olive oil in a large pot or Dutch oven over medium heat. Add onion, garlic, and bell pepper. Cook, stirring occasionally, until softened, about 5 minutes.
2. Add ground turkey and cook, breaking it up with a spoon, until browned. Drain any excess fat.
3. Stir in crushed tomatoes, black beans, pinto beans, diced tomatoes, chili powder, cumin, paprika, cayenne pepper (if using), and black pepper. Bring to a simmer.
4. Reduce heat and simmer for 20 minutes, stirring occasionally.
5. If desired, thicken the chili by mixing cornstarch with 2 tablespoons of water to form a slurry. Stir the slurry into the chili and cook for an additional minute, until thickened.
6. Taste and adjust seasonings as needed.
7. Serve hot, garnished with chopped fresh cilantro (optional).

Nutrition Information: Calories: 300-400, Fat: 10-15g, Cholesterol: 50mg, Protein: 30-40g, Fiber: 5-10g.

Tips:

- For a spicier chili, add more cayenne pepper or a chopped jalapeno pepper.
- You can add other vegetables to this chili, such as corn, carrots, or zucchini.
- If you don't have low-sodium chicken broth, you can use water instead.
- Serve the chili with your favorite toppings, such as low-fat cheese, avocado, salsa, or sour cream (use sparingly on the No Gallbladder Diet).

Vegetable Lentil Soup

Cooking Time: 30 minutes | **Prep Time**: 10 minutes | **Total Time**: 40 minutes | **Serving Size**: 4-6

Ingredients:

- 1 tablespoon olive oil
- 1 onion, chopped
- 2 celery stalks, chopped
- 2 carrots, chopped
- 2 cloves garlic, minced
- 1 teaspoon ground cumin
- 1/2 teaspoon ground turmeric
- 1/4 teaspoon black pepper
- 4 cups vegetable broth, low-sodium
- 1 cup brown lentils, rinsed
- 4 cups chopped mixed vegetables (such as zucchini, broccoli, potatoes, green beans)
- 1 (14.5 oz) can diced tomatoes, undrained
- 1/2 cup chopped fresh parsley
- Salt to taste (optional)

Directions:

1. Heat olive oil in a large pot over medium heat. Add onion, celery, and carrots and cook for 5 minutes, until softened.
2. Add garlic, cumin, turmeric, and black pepper. Cook for 1 minute, stirring constantly, until fragrant.
3. Add vegetable broth, lentils, and mixed vegetables. Bring to a boil, then reduce heat and simmer for 20 minutes, or until lentils are tender.
4. Stir in diced tomatoes and parsley. Cook for an additional 5 minutes, or until heated through.
5. Season with salt to taste, if desired.

Nutrition Information: Calories: 220, Fat: 4g, Saturated Fat: 1g, Cholesterol: 0mg, Sodium: 400mg, Fiber: 8g, Protein: 12g

Tips:

- For a smoother soup, puree about half of the soup using an immersion blender or food processor.
- Add other vegetables you like, such as bell peppers, spinach, or kale.
- Use cooked chicken breast or fish for added protein.
- Serve with a side of whole-wheat bread or brown rice for a complete meal.

Tomato Basil Soup

Cooking Time: 25 minutes | **Prep Time**: 10 minutes | **Total Time**: 35 minutes | **Serving Size**: 4

Ingredients:

- 1 tablespoon olive oil
- 1 onion, diced
- 2 cloves garlic, minced
- 1 (28-ounce) can crushed tomatoes
- 4 cups vegetable broth
- 1/2 teaspoon dried basil
- 1/4 teaspoon dried oregano
- Salt and pepper to taste
- 1/4 cup chopped fresh basil (optional)

Directions:

1. Heat olive oil in a large pot over medium heat. Add onion and cook until softened, about 5 minutes.
2. Add garlic and cook for an additional minute, until fragrant.
3. Stir in crushed tomatoes, vegetable broth, basil, oregano, salt, and pepper. Bring to a boil, then reduce heat and simmer for 20 minutes.
4. Remove from heat and allow to cool slightly.
5. Puree soup in a blender or food processor until smooth.
6. Return soup to pot and heat through.
7. Stir in chopped fresh basil, if using.
8. Serve immediately.

Nutrition Information: Calories: 180, Fat: 5g, Carbohydrates: 20g, Fiber: 3g, Protein: 5g

Tips:

- For a richer flavor, you can add a tablespoon of tomato paste along with the crushed tomatoes.
- If you don't have fresh basil, you can use 1/2 teaspoon of dried basil instead.
- You can also add other vegetables to this soup, such as carrots, celery, or zucchini.
- If you have a sensitive stomach, you may want to remove the skins from the tomatoes before adding them to the soup.

Potato Leek Soup

Cooking Time: 30 minutes | **Prep Time**: 10 minutes | **Total Time**: 40 minutes | **Serving Size**: 4

Ingredients:

- 1 tablespoon olive oil
- 1 leek, white and light green parts only, thinly sliced
- 2 cloves garlic, minced
- 4 cups vegetable broth
- 2 pounds russet potatoes, peeled and diced
- 1/2 teaspoon dried thyme
- 1/4 teaspoon salt
- 1/4 teaspoon black pepper
- 1/4 cup chopped fresh parsley (optional)

Directions:

1. Heat olive oil in a large pot or Dutch oven over medium heat. Add leek and cook, stirring occasionally, until softened, about 5 minutes. Add garlic and cook for an additional minute, until fragrant.
2. Add vegetable broth, potatoes, thyme, salt, and pepper to the pot. Bring to a boil, then reduce heat and simmer for 20 minutes, or until potatoes are tender.
3. Remove from heat and let cool slightly. Using an immersion blender or blender, puree soup until smooth. You can also mash the potatoes with a potato masher for a chunkier soup.
4. Taste and adjust seasonings as needed. Serve hot, garnished with fresh parsley (optional).

Nutrition Information: Calories: 220, Fat: 6g, Saturated Fat: 2g, Cholesterol: 0mg, Sodium: 400mg, Carbohydrates: 30g, Fiber: 5g, Protein: 5g

Tips:

- For a richer flavor, you can use a combination of olive oil and butter to cook the leek and garlic.
- If you don't have vegetable broth, you can use chicken broth or water. However, chicken broth may not be suitable for a no gallbladder diet, so check with your doctor first.
- You can add other vegetables to this soup, such as carrots, celery, or green beans.
- If you find the soup is too thick, you can add more broth or water to thin it out.
- To make this soup ahead of time, let it cool completely and then store it in the refrigerator for up to 3 days. Reheat gently over low heat before serving.

Minestrone Soup

Cooking Time: 30 minutes | **Prep Time**: 15 minutes | **Total Time**: 45 minutes | **Servings**: 4-6

Ingredients:

- 1 tablespoon olive oil
- 1 small onion, chopped
- 2 carrots, chopped
- 2 celery stalks, chopped
- 1 clove garlic, minced
- 4 cups low-sodium vegetable broth
- 1 (14.5 oz) can diced tomatoes, undrained
- 1 (15 oz) can cannellini beans, drained and rinsed
- 1 cup chopped zucchini
- 1/2 cup frozen peas
- 1/4 cup chopped fresh parsley
- Salt and pepper to taste

Directions:

1. Heat olive oil in a large pot over medium heat. Add onion, carrots, and celery and cook until softened, about 5 minutes.
2. Add garlic and cook for another minute, until fragrant.
3. Pour in vegetable broth and diced tomatoes. Bring to a boil, then reduce heat and simmer for 15 minutes.
4. Add cannellini beans, zucchini, and peas. Simmer for another 10 minutes, or until vegetables are tender.
5. Stir in parsley and season with salt and pepper to taste.
6. Serve hot and enjoy!

Nutrition Information: Calories: 200, Fat: 5g, Saturated Fat: 1g, Cholesterol: 0mg, Sodium: 400mg, Carbohydrates: 30g, Fiber: 5g, Protein: 10g

Tips:
- For a richer flavor, you can add a tablespoon of chopped fresh herbs like basil or oregano along with the parsley.
- If you don't have vegetable broth, you can use low-sodium chicken broth instead. Just be mindful of the added sodium content.
- To make this soup even more filling, you can add cooked pasta, quinoa, or brown rice.
- You can also adjust the vegetables to your liking. Other good options include green beans, corn, or chopped spinach.
- Make sure to cool the soup slightly before serving, especially if you have sensitive digestion.

Vegetable Quinoa Soup

Cooking Time: 30 minutes | **Prep Time**: 10 minutes | **Total Time**: 40 minutes | **Serving Size**: 4-6

Ingredients:

- 1 tablespoon olive oil
- 1 onion, diced
- 2 carrots, diced
- 2 celery stalks, diced
- 2 cloves garlic, minced
- 4 cups vegetable broth
- 1 cup chopped zucchini
- 1 cup chopped broccoli florets
- 1/2 cup chopped green beans
- 1/2 cup quinoa, rinsed
- 1 teaspoon dried oregano
- 1/2 teaspoon salt
- 1/4 teaspoon black pepper
- 1/4 cup chopped fresh parsley, for garnish (optional)

Directions:

1. Heat olive oil in a large pot over medium heat. Add onion, carrots, and celery and cook until softened, about 5 minutes.
2. Add garlic and cook for another minute, until fragrant.
3. Add vegetable broth, zucchini, broccoli, green beans, quinoa, oregano, salt, and pepper. Bring to a boil, then reduce heat and simmer for 20 minutes, or until quinoa is cooked through and vegetables are tender.
4. Remove from heat and garnish with fresh parsley, if desired.

Nutrition Information: Calories: 250, Fat: 4g, Fiber: 5g, Protein: 10g, Carbohydrates: 30g

Tips:

- For a thicker soup, mash some of the cooked vegetables with a fork before serving.
- You can add other vegetables to this soup, such as chopped mushrooms, spinach, or kale.
- If you don't have vegetable broth, you can use low-sodium chicken broth instead.
- Serve with a side of whole-wheat bread or crackers for a complete meal.

Mushroom Barley Soup

Prep time: 10 minutes | **Cooking time**: 30 minutes | **Total time**: 40 minutes | **Serving Size**: 4

Ingredients:

- 1 tablespoon olive oil
- 1 onion, chopped
- 2 carrots, chopped
- 2 celery stalks, chopped
- 4 cloves garlic, minced
- 4 cups vegetable broth
- 1 cup pearl barley
- 8 ounces sliced mushrooms (cremini, Portobello, or a mix)
- 1 teaspoon dried thyme
- 1/2 teaspoon dried rosemary
- Salt and pepper to taste
- 1/4 cup chopped fresh parsley, for garnish (optional)

Directions:

1. Heat the olive oil in a large pot or Dutch oven over medium heat. Add the onion, carrots, and celery and cook, stirring occasionally, until softened, about 5 minutes.
2. Add the garlic and cook for another minute, until fragrant.
3. Stir in the vegetable broth, barley, mushrooms, thyme, and rosemary. Bring to a boil, then reduce heat and simmer for 30 minutes, or until the barley is tender and the soup has thickened slightly.
4. Season with salt and pepper to taste. Garnish with fresh parsley, if desired.

Nutrition Information: Calories: 220, Fat: 4g, Saturated fat: 1g, Cholesterol: 0mg, Carbohydrates: 32g, Fiber: 8g, Protein: 10g

Tips:

- You can use any type of mushrooms you like in this soup. If you're using wild mushrooms, be sure to clean them thoroughly.
- For a richer flavor, you can sauté the mushrooms in a separate pan with a little butter or olive oil before adding them to the soup.
- If you don't have fresh herbs, you can use 1/2 teaspoon dried thyme and 1/4 teaspoon dried rosemary instead.
- To make this soup even more filling, you can add cooked chicken or shredded leftover turkey.
- Leftovers can be stored in the refrigerator for up to 3 days or frozen for up to 3 months.

Grilled Lemon Herb Chicken Breast

Cooking Time: 20-25 minutes | **Prep Time**: 10 minutes | **Total Time**: 30-35 minutes | **Serving Size**: 2

Ingredients:

- 2 boneless, skinless chicken breasts
- 1/4 cup olive oil
- 2 tablespoons lemon juice
- 1 teaspoon dried oregano
- 1/2 teaspoon dried thyme
- 1/4 teaspoon garlic powder
- 1/4 teaspoon black pepper
- Pinch of salt (optional, adjust based on your individual needs)
- Fresh lemon wedges, for serving (optional)

Directions:

1. Marinate: In a shallow dish, whisk together olive oil, lemon juice, oregano, thyme, garlic powder, pepper, and salt (if using). Place chicken breasts in the marinade, turning to coat evenly. Cover and refrigerate for at least 30 minutes, or up to 4 hours for more intense flavor.
2. Preheat Grill: Preheat your grill to medium-high heat. If using a charcoal grill, ensure the coals are white-hot with little to no flame.
3. Grill Chicken: Remove chicken from marinade and discard any remaining marinade. Place chicken breasts on the preheated grill. Grill for 5-7 minutes per side, or until cooked through and juices run clear when an internal temperature thermometer inserted into the thickest part of the breast reaches 165°F. Avoid overcooking to prevent dryness.
4. Rest and Serve: Transfer chicken to a plate and let rest for 5 minutes before serving. This allows the juices to redistribute for a more tender and flavorful result. Serve with lemon wedges, if desired, and enjoy!

Nutrition Information: Calories: 250, Fat: 5g, Saturated Fat: 1g, Cholesterol: 70mg, Protein: 35g, Carbohydrates: 1g, Fiber: 0g, Sodium: 150mg

Tips:

- For a thicker marinade and additional flavor, add 1 tablespoon Dijon mustard to the marinade.
- If you don't have a grill, you can bake the chicken in a preheated oven at 400°F for 20-25 minutes, or until cooked through.
- Serve with grilled vegetables, roasted potatoes, or a light salad for a complete and balanced meal.
- Be mindful of individual sodium restrictions and adjust the amount of salt used in the recipe accordingly.

Baked Pesto Chicken Thighs

Cooking time: 25-30 minutes | **Prep time**: 10 minutes | **Total time**: 35-40 minutes | **Serving size**: 4

Ingredients:

- 4 bone-in, skinless chicken thighs (about 1.5 lbs.)
- 1/4 cup store-bought pesto (look for low-fat options or adjust based on your dietary needs)
- 1 tablespoon olive oil
- 1/2 teaspoon dried oregano
- 1/4 teaspoon garlic powder
- Pinch of salt and black pepper
- Optional: Cherry tomatoes, chopped bell peppers, sliced zucchini, other low-fat vegetables

Directions:

1. Preheat oven to 400°F (200°C). Line a baking sheet with parchment paper.
2. Pat chicken thighs dry and season with salt and pepper.
3. In a small bowl, mix olive oil, oregano, garlic powder, and pesto.
4. Spread pesto mixture evenly over chicken thighs. You can either coat the entire thigh or just the top for less fat content.
5. Arrange chicken thighs on the prepared baking sheet. Tuck any vegetables under or around the chicken if using.
6. Bake for 25-30 minutes, or until chicken is cooked through and juices run clear when pierced with a fork. An instant-read thermometer inserted into the thickest part of the thigh should reach 165°F (74°C).
7. Let cool slightly before serving.

Nutrition information: Varies depending on ingredients used. Estimate for 1 serving (with full-fat pesto and olive oil): Calories: 350, Protein: 30g, Fat: 25g, Carbohydrates: 5g

Tips:

- Choose lean chicken thighs and remove any visible fat. Skinless, boneless thighs might be a better option depending on your individual tolerance.
- Use low-fat pesto. Look for options made with olive oil instead of nuts or cheese.
- Limit oil and added fats. Reduce the amount of olive oil used or try substituting with low-fat cooking spray.
- Focus on vegetables. Add low-fat vegetables like cherry tomatoes, zucchini, or bell peppers for additional nutrients and flavor.
- Consult a healthcare professional for personalized guidance. They can adjust the recipe based on your specific needs and restrictions.

Slow Cooker Chicken and Vegetable Stew

Cooking Time: 4-6 hours on low, or 2-3 hours on high | **Prep Time**: 15 minutes | **Total Time**: 4 hours 15 minutes - 8 hours 15 minutes | **Serving Size**: 4-6

Ingredients:

- 1 tablespoon olive oil
- 1 pound boneless, skinless chicken breasts or thighs, trimmed and cut into bite-sized pieces
- 1 onion, chopped
- 2 carrots, chopped
- 2 celery stalks, chopped
- 2 cloves garlic, minced
- 4 cups low-sodium chicken broth
- 1 (14.5-ounce) can diced tomatoes, undrained
- 1/2 cup chopped green beans
- 1/2 cup frozen peas
- 1/4 cup chopped fresh parsley
- 1 teaspoon dried thyme
- 1/2 teaspoon dried rosemary
- Salt and black pepper to taste

Directions:

1. Heat olive oil in a large skillet over medium heat. Add chicken and cook until golden brown on all sides. Remove from pan and set aside.
2. Add onion, carrots, and celery to the pan and cook until softened, about 5 minutes. Add garlic and cook for an additional minute, until fragrant.
3. Transfer vegetables to the slow cooker along with cooked chicken, chicken broth, diced tomatoes, green beans, peas, parsley, thyme, and rosemary. Season with salt and pepper to taste.
4. Cover the slow cooker and cook on low for 4-6 hours, or on high for 2-3 hours, or until chicken is cooked through and vegetables are tender.
5. Serve immediately, garnished with additional fresh parsley if desired.

Nutrition Information: Calories: 350-400, Fat: 10-15g, Saturated Fat: 3-5g, Cholesterol: 50mg, Carbohydrates: 30-35g, Fiber: 5-7g, Protein: 30-35g

Tips:

- You can use boneless, skinless chicken thighs instead of breasts for added flavor and juiciness.
- Feel free to add other vegetables to the stew, such as potatoes, zucchini, or corn.
- If you prefer a thicker stew, whisk together 1 tablespoon cornstarch with 2 tablespoons water in a small bowl and stir it into the stew during the last 15 minutes of cooking.
- For a richer flavor, use bone-in, skin-on chicken thighs and remove the skin before serving. However, remember that this will increase the cholesterol content.
- If you have specific gallbladder diet restrictions, consult your doctor or a registered dietitian before consuming this recipe.

Chicken and Vegetable Stir-Fry

Cooking Time: 15 minutes | **Prep Time**: 10 minutes | **Total Time**: 25 minutes | **Serving Size**: 2

Ingredients:

- 1 tablespoon avocado oil
- 1 pound boneless, skinless chicken breasts, thinly sliced
- 1/2 onion, thinly sliced
- 1 red bell pepper, thinly sliced
- 1 green bell pepper, thinly sliced
- 1 cup broccoli florets
- 1/2 cup sugar snap peas
- 1/4 cup low-sodium chicken broth
- 1 tablespoon cornstarch
- 1/4 teaspoon ground ginger
- 1/8 teaspoon garlic powder
- Salt and pepper to taste
- 1/4 cup chopped fresh cilantro, for garnish (optional)
- 1/4 avocado, thinly sliced (optional)

Directions:

1. Heat avocado oil in a large skillet or wok over medium-high heat. Add chicken and cook until browned and cooked through, about 5 minutes. Remove from pan and set aside.
2. Add onion, bell peppers, and broccoli to the pan. Cook for 5 minutes, or until softened.
3. Add sugar snap peas and cook for an additional 2 minutes.
4. In a small bowl, whisk together chicken broth, cornstarch, ginger, and garlic powder.
5. Return chicken to the pan and pour in the broth mixture. Cook for 1-2 minutes, or until sauce thickens and bubbles.
6. Season with salt and pepper to taste.
7. Serve immediately, garnished with cilantro and avocado (if using).

Nutrition Information: Calories: 350, Fat: 12g, Saturated Fat: 2g, Cholesterol: 70mg, Carbohydrates: 25g, Fiber: 5g, Sugar: 5g, Protein: 30g

Tips:

- You can use boneless, skinless chicken thighs instead of breasts.
- Feel free to add other vegetables to this stir-fry, such as carrots, snow peas, or mushrooms.
- If you don't have cornstarch, you can thicken the sauce with a slurry made from 1 tablespoon of water and 1 tablespoon of arrowroot powder.
- Serve this stir-fry over brown rice, quinoa, or noodles.

Grilled Honey Mustard Chicken Skewers

Cooking Time: 15-20 minutes | **Prep Time**: 10 minutes | **Total Time**: 25-30 minutes | **Serving Size**: 4

Ingredients:

- 1 pound boneless, skinless chicken breasts, cut into bite-sized pieces
- 1/4 cup low-fat yogurt
- 2 tablespoons Dijon mustard
- 1 tablespoon honey
- 1 tablespoon olive oil
- 1/2 teaspoon dried thyme
- 1/4 teaspoon garlic powder
- 1/4 teaspoon onion powder
- Salt and pepper to taste
- Wooden skewers, soaked in water for at least 30 minutes

Directions:

1. In a large bowl, whisk together yogurt, Dijon mustard, honey, olive oil, thyme, garlic powder, onion powder, salt, and pepper.
2. Add chicken pieces to the marinade and toss to coat evenly. Cover and refrigerate for at least 30 minutes, or up to 4 hours.
3. Preheat your grill to medium-high heat.
4. Thread chicken pieces onto soaked skewers, leaving some space between each piece.
5. Grill the skewers for 5-7 minutes per side, or until the chicken is cooked through and reaches an internal temperature of 165°F. Brush with any remaining marinade during the last few minutes of grilling.
6. Serve immediately with your favorite side dishes, such as grilled vegetables, roasted potatoes, or a salad.

Nutrition Information: Calories: 250, Fat: 8g, Saturated Fat: 2g, Cholesterol: 70mg, Protein: 35g, Carbohydrates: 5g, Fiber: 1g, Sugar: 4g

Tips:

- Use lean cuts of chicken, such as chicken breasts or thighs without skin.
- Marinate the chicken for longer for more flavorful results.
- If you don't have Dijon mustard, you can use yellow mustard instead.
- Avoid using processed sugars like white sugar or brown sugar. Honey is a natural sweetener that is tolerated better in the No Gallbladder Diet.
- Be mindful of portion sizes and avoid overeating, even if the dish is healthy.
- Consult your doctor or a registered dietitian for personalized dietary advice.

Baked Chicken Parmesan

Prep Time: 20 minutes | **Cooking Time**: 25 minutes | **Total Time**: 45 minutes | **Serving Size**: 4

Ingredients:

- 4 boneless, skinless chicken breasts (thinly pounded)
- 1/4 cup all-purpose flour
- 1/2 teaspoon dried oregano
- 1/4 teaspoon garlic powder
- 1/4 teaspoon black pepper
- 1/2 cup fat-free or low-fat buttermilk
- 1/2 cup whole wheat breadcrumbs
- 1/4 cup grated Parmesan cheese
- 1/4 cup shredded part-skim mozzarella cheese
- 1/4 cup marinara sauce (low-fat or sugar-free option recommended)

Directions:

1. Preheat oven to 400°F (200°C). Line a baking sheet with parchment paper.
2. In a shallow dish, combine flour, oregano, garlic powder, and pepper. Dredge each chicken breast in the flour mixture, coating evenly.
3. Dip each coated chicken breast in the buttermilk, then coat with the breadcrumb mixture, pressing gently to adhere.
4. Place coated chicken breasts on the prepared baking sheet. Drizzle lightly with olive oil or cooking spray.
5. Bake for 20-25 minutes, or until chicken is cooked through and golden brown.
6. Top each chicken breast with a spoonful of marinara sauce, then sprinkle with Parmesan and mozzarella cheese.
7. Broil for 2-3 minutes, or until cheese is melted and bubbly.
8. Serve immediately with a side of pasta (whole-wheat recommended) or roasted vegetables.

Nutrition Information: Calories: 350, Fat: 12g, Saturated Fat: 4g, Cholesterol: 80mg, Sodium: 400mg, Carbohydrates: 30g, Fiber: 2g, Sugar: 5g, Protein: 40g

Tips:

- For added flavor, marinate the chicken in Italian dressing or a mixture of olive oil, lemon juice, and herbs for 30 minutes before coating.
- Use a nonstick cooking spray to coat the chicken instead of olive oil for further fat reduction.
- Experiment with different low-fat cheese options, such as feta or goat cheese.
- Serve with a side salad for a more balanced meal.

Lemon Garlic Chicken Pasta

Cooking Time: 20 minutes | **Prep Time**: 10 minutes | **Total Time**: 30 minutes | **Servings**: 2

Ingredients:

- 4 ounces boneless, skinless chicken breast, thinly sliced
- 1 tablespoon olive oil
- 2 cloves garlic, minced
- 1/4 teaspoon dried oregano
- Pinch of red pepper flakes (optional)
- 1/4 cup chicken broth
- 1/4 cup lemon juice
- 1 tablespoon grated lemon zest
- 1/4 cup chopped fresh parsley
- 4 ounces whole-wheat pasta (such as penne, rotini, or fusilli)
- Salt and freshly ground black pepper, to taste

Directions:

1. Prepare the chicken: Season the chicken breast slices with salt and pepper.
2. Cook the chicken: Heat olive oil in a large skillet over medium heat. Add the chicken and cook for 5-7 minutes per side, or until golden brown and cooked through. Remove the chicken from the pan and set aside.
3. Make the sauce: Reduce the heat to low and add the garlic, oregano, and red pepper flakes (if using) to the pan. Cook for 30 seconds, until fragrant.
4. Deglaze the pan: Add the chicken broth, lemon juice, and lemon zest to the pan. Scrape up any browned bits from the bottom of the pan.
5. Simmer the sauce: Bring the sauce to a simmer and cook for 5 minutes, or until slightly thickened.
6. Cook the pasta: While the sauce simmers, cook the pasta according to package directions. Drain the pasta, reserving 1/4 cup of the pasta water.
7. Assemble the dish: Add the cooked pasta, reserved pasta water, and chopped parsley to the pan with the sauce. Toss to combine.
8. Serve: Return the chicken to the pan and toss with the pasta and sauce. Serve immediately, garnished with additional fresh parsley (optional).

Nutrition Information: Calories: 400, Fat: 10g (Saturated Fat: 2g), Cholesterol: 70mg, Sodium: 300mg, Carbohydrates: 40g (Fiber: 4g), Protein: 30g

Tips:

- Use low-sodium chicken broth for a heart-healthy option.
- You can add other vegetables to this dish, such as broccoli florets, chopped spinach, or cherry tomatoes.
- If you don't have fresh parsley, you can substitute 1 teaspoon dried parsley.
- For a richer flavor, you can add a tablespoon of grated Parmesan cheese to the finished dish.

Chicken and Vegetable Curry

Cooking Time: 30 minutes | **Prep Time**: 10 minutes | **Total Time**: 40 minutes | **Serving Size**: 4

Ingredients:

- 1 tablespoon olive oil
- 1 medium onion, chopped
- 2 cloves garlic, minced
- 1 teaspoon ground ginger
- 1/2 teaspoon turmeric
- 1/4 teaspoon cumin
- 1/4 teaspoon coriander
- 1/4 teaspoon chili powder (optional)
- 1 (14.5-ounce) can diced tomatoes, undrained
- 1 (13.5-ounce) can light coconut milk
- 1 cup low-fat chicken broth
- 1 pound boneless, skinless chicken breasts, trimmed and cut into bite-sized pieces
- 1 cup mixed vegetables (such as broccoli, carrots, bell peppers)
- 1/4 cup chopped fresh cilantro
- Salt and pepper to taste

Directions:

1. Heat olive oil in a large pot or Dutch oven over medium heat. Add onion and cook until softened, about 5 minutes. Stir in garlic, ginger, turmeric, cumin, coriander, and chili powder (if using). Cook for 1 minute, stirring constantly.
2. Add diced tomatoes, coconut milk, and chicken broth. Bring to a simmer and cook for 5 minutes.
3. Add chicken pieces and simmer for 15-20 minutes, or until chicken is cooked through.
4. Stir in mixed vegetables and cook for an additional 5 minutes, or until tender-crisp.
5. Remove from heat and stir in cilantro. Season with salt and pepper to taste.
6. Serve immediately over brown rice or quinoa.

Nutrition Information: Calories: 300, Fat: 10g, Saturated Fat: 2g, Cholesterol: 50mg, Protein: 30g, Carbohydrates: 20g, Fiber: 5g

Tips:

- For a spicier curry, add a pinch of red pepper flakes or a chopped jalapeno pepper.
- You can substitute other low-fat protein sources, such as shrimp or tofu, for the chicken.
- If you don't have fresh cilantro, you can use 1 teaspoon dried cilantro.
- To make this recipe ahead of time, simply prepare the curry as instructed and store it in the refrigerator for up to 3 days. Reheat gently before serving.

Chicken Caesar Salad Wraps

Cooking Time: 20 minutes | **Prep Time**: 10 minutes | **Total Time**: 30 minutes | **Serving Size**: 2

Ingredients:

- 2 boneless, skinless chicken breasts
- 4 cups romaine lettuce, chopped
- 1/2 cup shredded Parmesan cheese
- 1/4 cup Caesar salad dressing (look for a low-fat version made with olive oil)
- 2 whole wheat tortillas
- Salt and pepper to taste

Directions:

1. To poach the chicken, bring a large pot of water to a simmer. Season the water with salt and pepper. Add the chicken breasts and cook for 15-20 minutes, or until cooked through. Remove from the water and let cool slightly.
2. Shred the chicken breasts with two forks.
3. In a large bowl, combine the romaine lettuce, Parmesan cheese, and Caesar dressing. Toss to coat.
4. Warm the tortillas in a microwave or dry skillet.
5. Divide the chicken and salad mixture between the tortillas. Wrap tightly and serve.

Nutrition Information: Calories: 350, Fat: 10g, Saturated Fat: 3g, Cholesterol: 70mg, Sodium: 350mg, Carbohydrates: 15g, Fiber: 2g, Protein: 35g

Tips:

- For a more flavorful chicken, add a few herbs and spices to the poaching water, such as thyme, rosemary, or bay leaves.
- If you don't have Parmesan cheese, you can use another type of hard cheese, such as Romano or Asia go.
- You can also add other toppings to your wraps, such as sliced avocado, cherry tomatoes, or cucumbers.
- Be sure to use a low-fat Caesar dressing that is made with olive oil. Avoid dressings that are high in saturated fat or added sugars.
- If you have any concerns about following a no-gallbladder diet, be sure to talk to your doctor or a registered dietitian.

Poached Salmon with Lemon Dill Sauce

Cooking Time: 10-12 minutes | **Prep Time**: 5 minutes | **Total Time**: 15-17 minutes | **Serving Size**: 2

Ingredients:

- 2 salmon fillets (6 oz each)
- 4 cups water
- 1 tablespoon lemon juice
- 1 teaspoon chopped fresh dill
- 1/2 teaspoon salt
- 1/4 teaspoon black peppercorns

For the sauce:

- 1/4 cup low-fat yogurt
- 1 tablespoon chopped fresh dill
- 1 tablespoon lemon juice
- Salt and pepper to taste

Directions:

1. In a large pot, bring water, lemon juice, dill, salt, and peppercorns to a simmer.
2. Gently add the salmon fillets to the simmering water. Cover and cook for 10-12 minutes, or until the salmon is cooked through and flakes easily with a fork.
3. While the salmon is cooking, prepare the sauce by whisking together yogurt, dill, lemon juice, salt, and pepper in a small bowl.
4. Remove salmon from the poaching liquid and flake it onto plates. Drizzle with the lemon dill sauce and enjoy.

Nutrition Information: Calories: 250, Protein: 32g, Fat: 8g, Saturated Fat: 2g, Carbohydrates: 2g, Fiber: 1g, Cholesterol: 60mg

Tips:

- To further reduce fat intake, choose wild-caught salmon over farm-raised.
- Avoid adding additional fatty ingredients like butter or cream cheese.
- Experiment with different herbs and spices to personalize the flavor.

Tilapia

Prep Time: 10 minutes | **Cooking Time**: 15 minutes | **Total Time**: 25 minutes | **Servings**: 2

Ingredients:

- 2 tilapia fillets (skinless and boneless)
- 1 tablespoon olive oil
- 1/2 teaspoon lemon juice
- 1/4 teaspoon dried thyme
- 1/4 teaspoon garlic powder
- Salt and black pepper to taste
- Optional: Chopped fresh herbs (dill, parsley, chives) for garnish

Directions:

1. Preheat oven to 400°F (200°C). Line a baking sheet with parchment paper for easy cleanup.
2. Pat the tilapia fillets dry with paper towels. This helps ensure even browning and crisping.
3. In a small bowl, whisk together olive oil, lemon juice, thyme, garlic powder, salt, and pepper.
4. Brush the tilapia fillets with the herb mixture, coating them evenly.
5. Place the tilapia fillets on the prepared baking sheet. Ensure they are not crowded, as this can affect cooking time and evenness.
6. Bake for 15 minutes, or until the tilapia is cooked through and flakes easily with a fork. The internal temperature should reach 145°F (63°C) for food safety.
7. Garnish with chopped fresh herbs (optional) and serve immediately with your choice of sides that adhere to the No Gallbladder Diet guidelines.

Nutritional Information: Calories: 180, Fat: 7g, Saturated Fat: 1g, Cholesterol: 50mg, Sodium: 180mg, Carbohydrates: 0g, Fiber: 0g, Sugar: 0g, Protein: 30g

Tips:

- Use low-fat or fat-free cooking methods like baking, poaching, or grilling to minimize fat intake.
- Avoid added fats like butter, margarine, or heavy cream sauces.
- Opt for lean protein sources like skinless and boneless fish, poultry, or lean cuts of meat.
- Choose low-fiber vegetables like carrots, green beans, or zucchini.
- Limit processed foods and opt for whole foods whenever possible.
- Consult a healthcare professional or registered dietitian for personalized guidance on managing your No Gallbladder Diet.

Poached Cod with Tomato and Basil:

Cooking Time: 10 minutes | **Prep Time**: 5 minutes | **Total Time**: 15 minutes | **Serving Size**: 1

Ingredients:

- 1 (4-ounce) cod fillet
- 1 cup low-sodium chicken broth
- 1/2 cup chopped tomatoes
- 1/4 cup chopped fresh basil
- 1/4 teaspoon salt
- 1/4 teaspoon black pepper

Directions:

1. In a large skillet, bring chicken broth to a simmer. Add cod fillet and cook for 5-7 minutes, or until cooked through.
2. Stir in tomatoes, basil, salt, and pepper. Cook for an additional 2-3 minutes, until tomatoes are heated through.
3. Serve immediately.

Nutritional Information: Calories: 150, Fat: 3g, Protein: 25g, Carbs: 5g

Tips

- Choose lean fish and seafood, such as salmon, cod, shrimp, and scallops.
- Avoid fried seafood and opt for baking, poaching, or grilling instead.
- Limit added fats and oils. Use olive oil in moderation and avoid butter, margarine, and other saturated fats.
- Eat plenty of fruits, vegetables, and whole grains for fiber and essential nutrients.
- Drink plenty of water throughout the day to stay hydrated.

Baked Trout with Lemon and Herbs

Cooking Time: 20 minutes | Prep **Time**: 5 minutes | **Total Time**: 25 minutes | **Serving Size**: 1

Ingredients:

- 1 trout fillet (skinless, boneless)
- 1/2 tablespoon olive oil
- 1/2 lemon, sliced
- 1/4 teaspoon dried thyme
- 1/4 teaspoon dried oregano
- Salt and black pepper to taste

Directions:

1. Preheat oven to 400°F (200°C). Line a baking sheet with foil.
2. Place the trout fillet on the prepared baking sheet. Drizzle with olive oil.
3. Top with lemon slices, thyme, and oregano. Season with salt and pepper.
4. Bake for 20 minutes, or until the fish is cooked through and flakes easily with a fork.
5. Serve immediately.

Nutritional Information: 180 calories, 30g protein, 4g fat (0.5g saturated fat), 0g carbs, 0g fiber

Tips:

- You can substitute other herbs for thyme and oregano, such as rosemary, basil, or dill.
- If you prefer a crispier skin, you can broil the fish for the last few minutes of cooking.
- Serve with roasted vegetables, quinoa, or brown rice for a complete meal.

Poached Trout with Lemon and Dill

Cooking Time: 10 minutes | Prep **Time**: 5 minutes | Total **Time**: 15 minutes | **Serving Size**: 1

Ingredients:

- 1 trout fillet (skinless, boneless)
- 4 cups water
- 1/2 lemon, sliced
- 1 sprig fresh dill
- Salt and black pepper to taste

Directions:

1. Bring the water to a simmer in a large pot.
2. Add the lemon slices and dill sprig.
3. Gently place the trout fillet in the simmering water.
4. Cover the pot and simmer for 10 minutes, or until the fish is cooked through and flakes easily with a fork.
5. Remove the fish from the pot and transfer to a plate.
6. Season with salt and pepper to taste.
7. Serve immediately.

Nutritional Information 170 calories, 28g protein, 2g fat (0.3g saturated fat), 0g carbs, 0g fiber

Tips:

- You can add other vegetables to the poaching liquid, such as carrots, celery, or onions.
- Serve with a squeeze of fresh lemon juice and a sprinkle of fresh dill.
- Use low-sodium broth instead of water for additional flavor.

Sardines

Cooking Time: 15 minutes | **Prep Time**: 5 minutes | **Total Time**: 20 minutes | **Serving Size**: 1

Ingredients:

- 4 fresh sardines, scaled and cleaned
- 1 tablespoon olive oil
- 1/2 lemon, juiced
- 1/4 teaspoon dried oregano
- 1/4 teaspoon garlic powder
- Salt and black pepper to taste
- Fresh herbs (optional): parsley, dill, or chives

Directions:

1. Preheat oven to 400°F (200°C). Line a baking sheet with parchment paper.
2. Pat the sardines dry with paper towels. Drizzle with olive oil and lemon juice.
3. In a small bowl, combine oregano, garlic powder, salt, and pepper. Season the sardines with the spice mixture, making sure to coat them evenly.
4. Arrange the sardines on the prepared baking sheet. Bake for 10-12 minutes, or until the flesh is opaque and flakes easily with a fork.
5. Garnish with fresh herbs (optional) and serve immediately.

Nutrition Information: Calories: 120, Fat: 6g, Saturated Fat: 1g, Cholesterol: 50mg, Sodium: 200mg, Protein: 15g

Tips:

- If you prefer a more hands-off approach, you can grill the sardines instead of baking them. Preheat your grill to medium-high heat and cook for 3-4 minutes per side, or until cooked through.
- To add more flavor, you can marinate the sardines in a mixture of olive oil, lemon juice, herbs, and spices for 30 minutes before cooking.
- Serve the sardines with roasted vegetables, quinoa, or brown rice for a complete and balanced meal.

Poached Mackerel with Vegetables

Cooking time: 15 minutes | **Prep time**: 5 minutes | **Total time**: 20 minutes | **Serving size**: 1

Ingredients:

- 1 mackerel fillet, skinless and boneless
- 1 cup water
- 1/2 onion, sliced
- 1 carrot, sliced
- 1 celery stalk, sliced
- 1/4 teaspoon dried parsley
- Salt and pepper to taste

Directions:

1. Bring the water to a simmer in a large saucepan.
2. Add the onion, carrot, celery, and parsley.
3. Season with salt and pepper.
4. Gently place the mackerel fillet in the simmering water.
5. Cover the pan and cook for 10-15 minutes, or until the fish is cooked through and flakes easily with a fork.
6. Remove the fish and vegetables from the pan and serve immediately.

Nutrition information: Calories: 150, Fat: 6g, Cholesterol: 40mg, Protein: 20g, Sodium: 150mg

Tips:

- Choose skinless and boneless mackerel fillets for easier preparation and digestion.
- Use low-fat cooking methods such as baking, poaching, or grilling.
- Avoid adding unhealthy fats such as butter, fried foods, or processed meats to your diet.
- Limit your intake of saturated and trans fats, which can worsen gallbladder symptoms.
- Talk to your doctor or a registered dietitian for personalized advice on managing your no-gallbladder diet.

Shrimp Base

Prep Time: 10 minutes | **Cooking Time**: 20 minutes | **Total Time**: 30 minutes | **Serving Size**: 4

Ingredients:

- 1 pound raw shrimp, peeled and deveined
- 1 onion, chopped
- 2 carrots, chopped
- 2 celery stalks, chopped
- 1 teaspoon dried thyme
- 1 bay leaf
- 1/2 teaspoon salt
- 1/4 teaspoon black pepper
- 6 cups water

Directions:

1. Rinse the shrimp and place them in a colander to drain.
2. In a large pot, heat 1 tablespoon of water over medium heat. Add the onion, carrots, and celery, and cook until softened, about 5 minutes.
3. Add the thyme, bay leaf, salt, and pepper to the pot. Cook for another minute.
4. Add the shrimp and water to the pot. Bring to a boil, then reduce heat and simmer for 15 minutes, or until the shrimp are cooked through.
5. Remove the pot from the heat and remove the bay leaf. Allow the shrimp base to cool slightly.
6. **For a smoother base:** Blend the shrimp base in a blender or food processor until desired consistency is reached. Strain if necessary.
7. Use the shrimp base immediately in your desired fish or seafood recipe. You can store leftovers in an airtight container in the refrigerator for up to 3 days.

Nutrition Information: Calories: 50, Fat: 1g, Protein: 9g, Carbohydrates: 2g

Tips:

- For a richer flavor, use a combination of shrimp shells and water instead of plain water. Discard the shells before blending.
- Adjust the seasonings to your taste. You can add a pinch of red pepper flakes for a bit of heat or a squeeze of lemon juice for brightness.
- Use this shrimp base for poaching fish, making seafood chowder, or adding flavor to pasta dishes.
- Remember, even though shrimp is generally low in fat, some individuals with gallbladder issues might still need to moderate their intake. Consult your doctor or a registered dietitian for personalized dietary advice.

Baked Scallops with Garlic and Parmesan

Cooking Time: 10 minutes | **Prep Time**: 5 minutes | **Total Time**: 15 minutes | **Serving Size**: 2-3

Ingredients:

- 12 sea scallops, rinsed and patted dry
- 1 tablespoon olive oil
- 2 cloves garlic, minced
- 1/4 cup breadcrumbs
- 1/4 cup grated Parmesan cheese
- 1 tablespoon chopped fresh parsley
- Pinch of salt and pepper

Directions:

1. Preheat oven to 400°F (200°C).
2. In a bowl, combine olive oil, garlic, breadcrumbs, Parmesan cheese, parsley, and a pinch of salt and pepper.
3. Arrange scallops in a single layer on a baking sheet. Top each scallop with the breadcrumb mixture.
4. Bake for 10 minutes, or until scallops are cooked through and breadcrumbs are golden brown.
5. Serve immediately.

Nutrition Information: Calories: 180, Fat: 8g, Protein: 23g, Carbohydrates: 2g

Tips

- Choose smaller scallops, as they are easier to digest.
- Avoid adding too much fat, such as fried scallops or creamy sauces.
- Opt for cooking methods like pan-searing, baking, or poaching instead of deep-frying.
- Use low-fat cooking oils like olive oil or canola oil.
- Experiment with different herbs and spices to add flavor without added fat.
- Always listen to your body and adjust the recipes as needed based on your individual tolerance.

Flounder

Cooking Time: 10-15 minutes | **Prep Time**: 10 minutes | **Total Time**: 20-25 minutes | **Serving Size**: 1

Ingredients

- 1 flounder fillet (skinless and boneless)
- 1 tablespoon olive oil or avocado oil
- 1/4 teaspoon dried thyme
- 1/4 teaspoon garlic powder
- Salt and pepper to taste
- 1/4 cup lemon juice (optional)
- Fresh herbs for garnish (optional)

Directions:

1. Preheat: Heat oil in a pan over medium heat. Alternatively, preheat oven to 400°F (200°C).
2. Season: Pat the flounder fillet dry and season with thyme, garlic powder, salt, and pepper.
3. Cook:
- Pan-frying: Add the flounder to the pan and cook for 4-5 minutes per side, or until golden brown and cooked through.
- Baking: Place the flounder on a baking sheet and bake for 15-20 minutes, or until cooked through.
4. Deglaze (optional): If pan-frying, remove the flounder from the pan and deglaze with lemon juice, scraping up any browned bits.
5. Serve: Plate the flounder and drizzle with the pan sauce (if using) or lemon juice (optional). Garnish with fresh herbs (optional).

Nutrition Information: Calories: 120-150, Fat: 3-5 grams, Protein: 20-25 grams, Carbohydrates: 0 grams

Tips:

- Choose lean fish: Flounder is a good choice as it's naturally low in fat.
- Limit added fat: Use a minimal amount of oil for cooking. Consider poaching or steaming the flounder for a fat-free option.
- Avoid rich sauces: Skip creamy sauces or gravies that are high in fat. Use lemon juice, herbs, or a light broth for flavor instead.
- Portion control: Stick to a single serving of fish to manage fat intake.
- Pair with healthy sides: Choose non-starchy vegetables like steamed broccoli, roasted asparagus, or a side salad with a light vinaigrette.

Haddock Poached in Tomato Broth

Cooking Time: 15 minutes | **Prep Time**: 10 minutes | **Total Time**: 25 minutes | **Serving Size**: 2

Ingredients:

- 2 (6-ounce) haddock fillets
- 1 (14.5-ounce) can diced tomatoes, undrained
- 1/2 cup low-sodium chicken broth
- 1/4 cup chopped fresh parsley
- 1 tablespoon lemon juice
- Salt and pepper to taste

Directions:

1. In a large saucepan, combine diced tomatoes, chicken broth, parsley, lemon juice, salt, and pepper.
2. Bring to a simmer over medium heat.
3. Add the haddock fillets and gently simmer for 15 minutes, or until the fish is cooked through and flakes easily with a fork.

Nutrition Information: Calories: 200, Protein: 25g, Fat: 3g, Carbohydrates: 5g

Tips:

- For both recipes, use skinless haddock fillets for easier digestion.
- Avoid using added fats, such as butter or oil, for cooking.
- You can add other vegetables to these recipes, such as steamed broccoli or carrots.
- Be sure to check the nutrition information of any packaged ingredients you use, as some may contain added sugars or unhealthy fats.

Fruit Salad

Prep Time: 10 minutes | **Cooking Time**: None | **Total Time**: 10 minutes | **Servings**: 2-3

Ingredients:

- 1 cup mixed berries (fresh or frozen)
- 1/2 cup diced pineapple
- 1/2 cup diced cantaloupe
- 1/4 cup seedless grapes, halved
- 1/4 cup chopped orange (remove white pith)
- 1 tablespoon chia seeds
- 1 tablespoon freshly squeezed orange juice
- 1/4 teaspoon ground cinnamon (optional)
- Mint leaves, for garnish (optional)

Directions:

1. Wash and prepare fruits: Thoroughly wash all fruits. Dice cantaloupe and pineapple, halve grapes, and segment orange, removing any white pith.
2. Combine fruits: In a bowl, gently combine mixed berries, pineapple, cantaloupe, grapes, and orange segments.
3. Add dressing: In a separate small bowl, whisk together orange juice, chia seeds, and cinnamon (if using). Pour dressing over the fruit mixture and toss gently to coat.
4. Chill and serve: Refrigerate the fruit salad for at least 15 minutes to allow the flavors to meld and chia seeds to plump. Garnish with mint leaves (optional) and serve chilled.

Nutrition Information: Calories: 120, Fat: 0.5g, Saturated Fat: 0g, Cholesterol: 0mg, Sodium: 5mg, Carbohydrates: 30g, Fiber: 4g, Sugar: 20g, Protein: 1g

Tips:

- For a richer flavor, use a squeeze of lime juice instead of orange juice.
- Add other no-gallbladder-friendly fruits like papaya, mango, or kiwi.
- If using frozen berries, thaw them slightly before adding to the salad.
- Make it a parfait! Layer the fruit salad with plain yogurt for a more substantial dessert.
- Top with toasted nuts or shredded coconut for added texture and flavor (if tolerated).
- Adjust the sweetness to your preference by adding a touch of honey or maple syrup.

Baked Apples

Cooking Time: 30-40 minutes | **Prep Time**: 10 minutes | **Total Time**: 40-50 minutes | **Serving Size**: 1

Ingredients

- 1 apple, firm and sweet variety like Gala or Honey crisp
- 1/4 teaspoon ground cinnamon
- 1/8 teaspoon ground nutmeg
- 1 tablespoon unsweetened applesauce
- 1/4 cup chopped walnuts or pecans (optional)
- 1 tablespoon dried cranberries or raisins (optional)
- 1/4 teaspoon maple syrup (optional)

Directions:

1. Preheat oven to 375°F (190°C).
2. Wash the apple and core it, leaving the bottom intact. You can use a melon baller or apple corer for this.
3. In a small bowl, combine cinnamon, nutmeg, and applesauce. Stir in chopped nuts and dried fruit (if using).
4. Fill the apple core with the prepared mixture. Drizzle with a touch of maple syrup (optional) for added sweetness.
5. Place the apple in a baking dish and bake for 30-40 minutes, or until the apple is tender and the filling is bubbly.
6. Let the apple cool slightly before serving. Enjoy!

Nutrition Information: Calories: 150, Fat: 2g, Cholesterol: 0mg, Sodium: 20mg, Carbohydrates: 30g, Fiber: 4g, Sugar: 20g (natural sugar from apples)

Tips:

- For a richer flavor, add a scoop of low-fat vanilla ice cream on top.
- To make this vegan, skip the honey and use agave syrup or date syrup instead.
- You can customize the filling with different spices or toppings like sliced banana, chopped dates, or a sprinkle of granola.
- Be mindful of portion sizes, as even small amounts of added sugar can still affect your digestion.

Greek Yogurt Parfait

Cooking Time: 0 minutes | **Prep Time**: 5 minutes | **Total Time**: 5 minutes | **Serving Size**: 1

Ingredients:

- 1/2 cup plain Greek yogurt (2% or non-fat)
- 1/4 cup fresh or frozen berries (such as blueberries, raspberries, strawberries)
- 1/4 cup sliced banana or other soft fruit
- 1/4 cup granola (choose a low-fat, low-sugar variety)
- 1 tablespoon chopped nuts or seeds (optional)
- 1 teaspoon honey or maple syrup (optional)
- Fresh mint sprig or other garnish (optional)

Directions:

1. Choose your ingredients: Select fruits that are low in fat and fiber, which can be difficult to digest after gallbladder removal. Avoid fatty nuts and seeds, and use granola sparingly. Opt for low-fat or non-fat yogurt.
2. Layer the parfait: In a glass or bowl, start with a layer of yogurt. Top with half of the berries and sliced fruit. Add half of the granola. Repeat with another layer of yogurt, fruit, and granola.
3. Customize: Drizzle with honey or maple syrup if desired. Top with chopped nuts or seeds for additional texture and flavor. Garnish with a fresh mint sprig or other herb for a refreshing touch.
4. Enjoy immediately: Parfaits are best enjoyed fresh, as the granola can become soggy if stored for too long.

Nutrition Information: Calories: 250-300, Fat: 5-10g, Carbohydrates: 20-30g, Protein: 15-20g, Fiber: 5-10g, Sugar: 5-10g

Tips:

- Use ripe, but not mushy, fruit.
- If using frozen fruit, thaw it slightly before layering.
- For a creamier texture, blend the yogurt with a touch of milk or almond milk before using.
- Experiment with different flavor combinations! Try other fruits, such as mango, papaya, or kiwi.
- Add a sprinkle of chia seeds or flaxseeds for an extra boost of omega-3 fatty acids.
- If you have concerns about specific ingredients, consult with your doctor or a registered dietitian for personalized guidance.

Chia Seed Pudding

Cooking Time: 5 minutes - 2 hours chilling (minimum) | **Prep Time**: 5 minutes | **Total Time**: 2 hours 5 minutes (minimum) | **Serving Size**: 1

Ingredients:

- 1/4 cup chia seeds
- 1 cup unsweetened plant-based milk (almond, coconut, oat, etc.)
- 1/4 cup mashed ripe banana, mango, or avocado (optional)
- 1/4 teaspoon vanilla extract
- 1/4 teaspoon ground cinnamon
- Pinch of stevia or monk fruit sweetener (optional)
- Fresh berries, chopped nuts, or shredded coconut for topping (optional)

Directions

1. Combine: In a jar or bowl, whisk together chia seeds, plant-based milk, mashed fruit (if using), vanilla extract, cinnamon, and sweetener (if using).
2. Chill: Cover the jar or bowl and refrigerate for at least 2 hours, or overnight for a thicker consistency. Stir occasionally during the first hour to prevent clumping.
3. Serve: Top with fresh berries, chopped nuts, or shredded coconut (optional). Enjoy!

Nutrition Information: Calories: 220, Fat: 8g (1g saturated), Carbohydrates: 22g (4g fiber, 7g sugar), Protein: 5g, Sodium: 30mg

Tips:

- For a richer flavor, use full-fat coconut milk or a combination of coconut milk and another plant-based milk.
- Add a pinch of turmeric or ginger for a warming twist.
- Experiment with different fruits and spices to create your own unique flavor combinations.
- If you prefer a warmer pudding, heat the plant-based milk before adding the chia seeds. However, note that chia seeds gel better when cold.
- Leftovers can be stored in the refrigerator for up to 3 days.

Banana Nice Cream

Cooking Time: None | **Prep Time**: 10 minutes | **Total Time**: 10 minutes | **Serving Size**: 1-2

Ingredients:

- 2 ripe bananas, frozen and chopped
- 1/2 cup unsweetened plant-based milk (almond, oat, or coconut milk work well)
- 1/4 teaspoon vanilla extract (optional)
- 1/4 cup optional add-ins (such as cocoa powder, peanut butter, chopped nuts, or berries)

Directions:

1. Prepare the bananas: Freeze the bananas for at least 4 hours, or overnight for best results. Chop them into smaller pieces before blending.
2. Blend the base: Combine the frozen bananas, plant-based milk, and vanilla extract (if using) in a high-powered blender. Blend until smooth and creamy, scraping down the sides as needed.
3. Add-ins (optional): If desired, stir in your chosen add-ins once the base is blended. Be careful not to over-blend, as this can melt the "nice cream."
4. Freeze and serve: Immediately transfer the "nice cream" to a container and freeze for at least 30 minutes to firm up. Enjoy!

Nutrition Information: Calories: 130-150, Fat: 2-3g, Carbohydrates: 25-30g, Fiber: 3-4g, Sugar: 15-20g, Protein: 1-2g

Tips:

- For a richer flavor, use very ripe bananas with brown spots.
- If your blender struggles, add a tablespoon of plant-based milk at a time until the mixture blends smoothly.
- Get creative with your add-ins! Experiment with different flavors and textures to find your perfect combination.
- This "nice cream" is best enjoyed immediately after freezing, as it can become icy if frozen for too long.
- If you have dietary restrictions, be sure to choose add-ins that are safe for your no gallbladder diet.

Rice Pudding

Prep Time: 10 minutes | **Cooking Time**: 45 minutes | **Total Time**: 55 minutes | **Serving Size**: 4

Ingredients

- 1 cup cooked white rice (Arborio or basmati recommended)
- 2 cups low-fat milk (almond, soy, or oat milk can be substituted)
- 1/4 cup water
- 1/4 cup sugar (or substitute with honey, maple syrup, or stevia)
- 1/2 teaspoon vanilla extract
- 1/4 teaspoon ground cinnamon
- Pinch of nutmeg
- Fresh fruit (optional, for topping)

Directions:

1. Prepare the rice: Cook the white rice according to package instructions and set aside to cool slightly.
2. Combine ingredients: In a medium saucepan, whisk together milk, water, sugar, vanilla extract, cinnamon, and nutmeg. Bring to a simmer over medium heat, whisking occasionally.
3. Add rice: Add the cooked rice to the simmering milk mixture and stir gently to combine. Reduce heat to low and simmer for 20 minutes, stirring occasionally, until rice is creamy and tender.
4. Thicken the pudding (optional): If you prefer a thicker pudding, whisk together 1 tablespoon cornstarch with 2 tablespoons cold water in a small bowl until smooth. Slowly whisk the cornstarch mixture into the simmering pudding and cook for an additional 2 minutes, stirring constantly, until thickened.
5. Cool and serve: Remove the pudding from the heat and let cool slightly. Divide the pudding among serving bowls and chill in the refrigerator for at least 1 hour before serving.
6. Top with fruit (optional): When serving, top the pudding with fresh fruit, such as berries, sliced peaches, or mangoes.

Nutrition Information: Calories: 220, Fat: 3g, Saturated Fat: 1g, Cholesterol: 0mg, Carbohydrates: 38g, Sugar: 18g, Fiber: 1g, Protein: 5g

Tips:

- For a richer flavor, use full-fat coconut milk instead of low-fat milk. However, keep in mind that this will increase the fat content per serving.
- Experiment with different spices, such as ginger, cardamom, or cloves, to add a unique flavor to your pudding.
- If you don't have a saucepan, you can make this rice pudding in the microwave. Simply combine all ingredients in a microwave-safe bowl and cook on high power for 3-4 minutes, stirring every minute, until heated through and thickened.
- Leftover rice pudding can be stored in the refrigerator for up to 3 days.

Coconut Macaroons

Cooking Time: 20 minutes | **Prep Time**: 10 minutes | **Total Time**: 30 minutes | **Serving Size:** 12

Ingredients:

- 1 cup unsweetened shredded coconut
- 1/2 cup almond flour
- 1/4 cup creamy almond butter
- 1/4 cup pure maple syrup
- 1/4 teaspoon vanilla extract
- 1/8 teaspoon sea salt

Directions:

1. Preheat oven to 350°F (175°C). Line a baking sheet with parchment paper.
2. In a large bowl, combine the shredded coconut, almond flour, and salt.
3. In a separate bowl, whisk together the almond butter, maple syrup, and vanilla extract until smooth.
4. Add the wet ingredients to the dry ingredients and mix well until a thick batter forms.
5. Roll the batter into 12 evenly sized balls. Place the balls on the prepared baking sheet, leaving space between them for spreading.
6. Bake for 20 minutes, or until the macaroons are golden brown and slightly firm to the touch.
7. Let the macaroons cool on the baking sheet for a few minutes before transferring them to a wire rack to cool completely.

Nutrition Information: Calories: 120, Fat: 8g, Carbohydrates: 10g, Fiber: 2g, Protein: 3g

Tips:

- For a richer flavor, use toasted coconut instead of unsweetened shredded coconut.
- If the batter is too dry, add a tablespoon of almond milk or water at a time until it reaches the desired consistency.
- You can dip the macaroons in melted dark chocolate for an extra decadent treat.
- Store the macaroons in an airtight container in the refrigerator for up to a week.

Pumpkin Pie Smoothie

Prep Time: 5 minutes | **Cooking Time**: None | **Total Time**: 5 minutes | **Serving Size**: 1

Ingredients:
- 1 cup unsweetened canned pumpkin puree
- 1 cup unsweetened almond milk
- 1/2 ripe banana, frozen
- 1/4 cup plain Greek yogurt (choose lactose-free if needed)
- 1/2 teaspoon ground cinnamon
- 1/4 teaspoon ground ginger
- 1/4 teaspoon ground nutmeg
- Pinch of ground cloves
- Optional: 1 tablespoon maple syrup or honey (choose low-glycemic option if needed)
- Optional: Ice cubes, for desired consistency

Directions:

1. Gather your ingredients: Make sure all ingredients are chilled for a thicker smoothie.
2. Combine in a blender: Add pumpkin puree, almond milk, frozen banana, Greek yogurt, spices, and optional sweetener to your blender.
3. Blend until smooth: Blend on high speed for about 30 seconds, or until desired consistency is reached. Add ice cubes gradually if you prefer a thicker smoothie.
4. Taste and adjust: If desired, add more sweetener or spices to taste.
5. Serve immediately: Enjoy your pumpkin pie smoothie as a refreshing and nutritious dessert or snack.

Nutrition Information: Calories: 250, Fat: 3g, Carbs: 35g, Fiber: 4g, Sugar: 18g, Protein: 5g

Tips:

- For a richer flavor, use homemade pumpkin puree.
- Substitute the banana with other frozen fruits like mango or pineapple.
- Add a scoop of protein powder for an extra boost of protein.
- Use unsweetened applesauce instead of the banana for a thicker and less sweet smoothie.
- Top your smoothie with a sprinkle of pumpkin seeds, chopped nuts, or a drizzle of cinnamon for added texture and flavor.

Oatmeal Cookies

Prep Time: 15 minutes | **Cooking Time**: 12-15 minutes | **Total Time**: 27-30 minutes | **Serving Size**: 12

Ingredients:

- 1 cup rolled oats
- 1/2 cup whole wheat flour
- 1/4 cup unsweetened applesauce
- 1/4 cup honey
- 1/4 cup mashed banana
- 1/4 cup chopped dried cranberries (optional)
- 1/4 cup chopped walnuts (optional)
- 1 teaspoon ground cinnamon
- 1/2 teaspoon baking powder
- 1/4 teaspoon baking soda
- 1/4 teaspoon salt

Directions:

1. Preheat oven to 375°F (190°C) and line a baking sheet with parchment paper.
2. In a large bowl, whisk together the oats, flour, cinnamon, baking powder, baking soda, and salt.
3. In a separate bowl, mash the banana and combine it with the applesauce, honey, and any desired chopped nuts and dried fruit.
4. Add the wet ingredients to the dry ingredients and mix until just combined. Do not over mix.
5. Drop rounded tablespoons of dough onto the prepared baking sheet.
6. Bake for 12-15 minutes, or until the edges are golden brown.
7. Let the cookies cool on the baking sheet for a few minutes before transferring them to a wire rack to cool completely.

Nutrition Information per cookie: Calories: 120, Fat: 3g (Saturated fat: 1g), Cholesterol: 0mg, Sodium: 70mg, Carbohydrates: 22g (Fiber: 3g) Sugar: 8g, Protein: 2g

Tips:

- For a chewier cookie, use less flour or add an extra tablespoon of mashed banana.
- You can substitute other dried fruits or nuts for the cranberries and walnuts, or omit them altogether.
- You can also use a combination of different flours, such as almond flour or oat flour.
- Make sure your mashed banana is very ripe for the best texture and sweetness.
- If you don't have applesauce, you can use mashed pear or pumpkin puree instead.
- These cookies can be stored in an airtight container at room temperature for up to 3 days.

Angel Food Cake with Berries

Cooking Time: 45 minutes | **Prep Time**: 15 minutes | **Total Time**: 60 minutes | **Serving Size**: 12

Ingredients:

- 1 1/2 cups granulated sugar
- 1 1/4 cups powdered sugar
- 1 1/2 teaspoons cream of tartar
- 12 large egg whites
- 1 teaspoon vanilla extract
- 1/4 teaspoon salt
- 1/2 cup unsweetened applesauce
- 1 teaspoon almond extract
- 1 cup fresh berries (such as strawberries, blueberries, raspberries)

Directions:

1. Preheat oven to 350°F (175°C). Grease and flour a 12-cup angel food cake pan.
2. In a large bowl, whisk together granulated sugar, powdered sugar, and cream of tartar.
3. In a separate bowl, beat egg whites with an electric mixer on high speed until stiff peaks form. Gradually add the sugar mixture to the egg whites, beating continuously until incorporated. Beat in vanilla extract and salt.
4. Gently fold in applesauce and almond extract into the egg white mixture until just combined.
5. Pour batter into the prepared pan and smooth the top. Bake for 45 minutes, or until a toothpick inserted into the center comes out clean.
6. Let the cake cool in the pan for 10 minutes, then invert onto a wire rack to cool completely.
7. Once cool, top with fresh berries and enjoy!

Nutrition Information: Calories: 100, Fat: 0g, Cholesterol: 0mg, Carbohydrates: 20g, Sugar: 15g, Protein: 3g

Tips:

- For a richer flavor, use almond flour instead of applesauce.
- You can also add 1/4 cup of chopped nuts to the batter.
- Make sure to use a clean, grease-free bowl when beating the egg whites. Any traces of fat can prevent them from whipping up properly.
- Don't over mix the batter once you add the applesauce and almond extract. Just gently fold them in until combined.
- If you don't have an angel food cake pan, you can use a Bundt pan or another tube pan. Just adjust the baking time accordingly.

MEAL PLANNING

WEEK 1

Day 1
Breakfast: Greek Yogurt Parfait
Lunch: Grilled Lemon Herb Chicken Salad
Dinner: Grilled Lemon Herb Chicken with Steamed Vegetables

Day 2
Breakfast: Oatmeal with Berries and Almonds
Lunch: Quinoa and Vegetable Stir-Fry
Dinner: Baked Salmon with Quinoa and Roasted Asparagus

Day 3
Breakfast: Smoothie Bowl
Lunch: Salmon and Avocado Wrap
Dinner: Turkey and Vegetable Stir-Fry

Day 4:
Breakfast: Whole Wheat Toast with Avocado and Poached Egg
Lunch: Turkey and Hummus Veggie Wrap
Dinner: Shrimp and Veggie Skewers with Brown Rice

Day 5:
Breakfast: Quinoa Breakfast Bowl
Lunch: Mediterranean Chickpea Salad
Dinner: Vegetarian Chili with Whole Grain Bread

Day 6:
Breakfast: Cottage Cheese Pancakes
Lunch: Vegetable and Lentil Soup
Dinner: Baked Cod with Lemon Garlic Butter Sauce and Steamed Green Beans

Day 7:
Breakfast: Vegetable Frittata
Lunch: Tuna and White Bean Salad
Dinner: Tofu Stir-Fry with Brown Rice

WEEK 2

Day 8:
Breakfast: Chia Seed Pudding
Lunch: Grilled Veggie and Chicken Kabobs
Dinner: Grilled Chicken Caesar Salad

Day 9:
Breakfast: Banana Almond Butter Toast
Lunch: Shrimp and Avocado Salad
Dinner: Quinoa Stuffed Bell Peppers

Day 10:
Breakfast: Egg Muffins
Lunch: Vegetable and Turkey Sauté
Dinner: Vegetable and Chickpea Curry with Cauliflower Rice

Day 11:
Breakfast: Yogurt and Fruit Smoothie
Lunch: Grilled Lemon Herb Chicken Salad
Dinner: Baked Salmon with Quinoa and Roasted Asparagus

Day 12:
Breakfast: Vegetable Omelette
Lunch: Quinoa and Vegetable Stir-Fry
Dinner: Turkey and Vegetable Stir-Fry

Day 13:
Breakfast: Buckwheat Pancakes
Lunch: Salmon and Avocado Wrap
Dinner: Shrimp and Veggie Skewers with Brown Rice

Day 14:
Breakfast: Salmon and Avocado Toast
Lunch: Mediterranean Chickpea Salad
Dinner: Vegetarian Chili with Whole Grain Bread

FREQUENTLY ASKED QUESTIONS (FAQS)

1. **What is a no gallbladder diet?** A no-gallbladder diet, also known as a post-cholecystectomy diet, is a food plan meant to assist persons who have had their gallbladder removed to control their digestion and reduce pain.

2. **Why do I need to maintain a particular diet after gallbladder removal?** The gallbladder contains bile, which assists in the digestion of lipids. After gallbladder removal, bile is continually pumped into the digestive system, which may occasionally contribute to digestive difficulties, particularly with fatty meals. Following a particular diet may help control these symptoms.

3. **What foods should I avoid on a no-gallbladder diet?** Foods to avoid often include high-fat meals, spicy foods, processed foods, carbonated drinks, caffeine, alcohol, and some fresh vegetables that may be difficult to digest.

4. **What foods can I consume on a no-gallbladder diet?** Foods that are typically well-tolerated on a no-gallbladder diet include lean proteins, low-fat dairy products, and healthy fats in moderation, fruits, vegetables, whole grains, and fiber-rich meals.

5. **How can I manage digestive symptoms on a no-gallbladder diet?** Managing digestive symptoms may involve eating smaller, more frequent meals; choosing low-fat options; avoiding trigger foods; staying hydrated; and gradually reintroducing foods into your diet while monitoring your body's response.

6. **Can I still eat sweets on a no-gallbladder diet?** Yes, there are many dessert alternatives that are good for persons on a no-gallbladder diet, including fruit-based sweets, yogurt-based delights, and desserts prepared with healthy grains and low-fat components.

7. **Should I take any vitamins on a no-gallbladder diet?** Some people may benefit from taking digestive enzyme supplements with meals to help in the digestion of lipids. However, it's vital to contact a healthcare practitioner before adding any supplements to your regimen.

8. **How can I plan meals on a no-gallbladder diet?** Meal planning on a no-gallbladder diet requires picking lean meats, adding lots of fruits and vegetables, choosing whole grains, opting for low-fat dairy products, and avoiding high-fat or spicy meals.

9. **Can I still enjoy eating out on a no-gallbladder diet?** Yes, you may still enjoy eating out while following a no-gallbladder diet by making careful choices, such as picking grilled or baked alternatives, asking for dressings and sauces on the side, and avoiding fried or excessively processed items.

10. **Is it possible to adapt to life without a gallbladder?** Yes, most individuals adapt well to life without a gallbladder by making dietary alterations, keeping hydrated, controlling stress, and adopting good lifestyle practices. However, it may take some time for your body to adjust properly.

GLOSSARY

1. **Gallbladder**: A tiny organ found underneath the liver that stores bile generated by the liver and releases it to help in the digestion of fats.

2. **Cholecystectomy**: Surgical removal of the gallbladder, commonly owing to gallstones, inflammation, or other gallbladder-related disorders.

3. **Bile**: A fluid generated by the liver that assists in the digestion and absorption of fats in the small intestine.

4. **Post-cholecystectomy**: Referring to the time after gallbladder removal.

5. **Digestive enzymes**: Proteins that help break down food into smaller molecules for absorption and usage by the body. Some people may take digestive enzyme supplements to help in the digestion of fats following gallbladder removal.

6. **Fiber**: A form of carbohydrate found in plant-based meals that supports digestive health, regulates bowel movements, and helps avoid constipation. Soluble fiber dissolves in water and creates a gel-like material, whereas insoluble fiber adds weight to feces.

7. **Lean proteins**: Protein foods that are low in fat, such as skinless chicken, fish, tofu, lentils, and lean cuts of meat.

8. **Healthy fats**: Unsaturated fats that are healthy for heart health, including monounsaturated fats found in foods like avocados, almonds, and olive oil, and polyunsaturated fats found in foods like fatty fish, flaxseeds, and walnuts.

9. **Whole grains**: Grains that maintain all portions of the grain kernel, including the bran, germ, and endosperm, giving fiber, vitamins, minerals, and other nutrients. Examples include brown rice, quinoa, oats, whole wheat bread, and barley.

10. **Spices**: Flavorful compounds produced from plants, seeds, fruits, or roots, typically used to season and improve the flavor of food. While spices may add taste to dishes, spicy foods may be unpleasant for some folks after gallbladder ectomy.

11. **Probiotics**: Beneficial microorganisms that support gut health and digestion. Probiotics may be found in fermented foods like yogurt, kefir, sauerkraut, and kimchi, as well as in supplement form.

12. **Hydration**: The process of delivering fluids to the body to maintain optimum fluid balance, assist digestion, and avoid dehydration. Adequate hydration is vital for general health, especially after gallbladder resection.

13. **Meal planning**: The act of scheduling meals and snacks in advance, often to fulfill nutritional objectives, manage health issues, or suit lifestyle choices. Meal planning may assist those on a no-gallbladder diet make healthful choices and avoid trigger foods.

14. **Dietitian**: A healthcare practitioner specialized in nutrition and dietetics who gives tailored nutrition advice and direction to clients to help them accomplish their health and wellness objectives, particularly those following a no-gallbladder diet.